- You can return this item to any Bournemouth library but not all libraries are open every day.
- Items must be returned on or before the due date. Please note that you will be charged for items returned late.
- Items may be renewed unless requested by another customer.
- Renewals can be made in any library, by telephone, email or online via the website. Your membership card number and PIN will be required.
- Please look after this item - you may be charged for any damage.

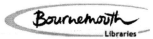

Bournemouth
Libraries

www.bournemouth.gov.uk/libraries

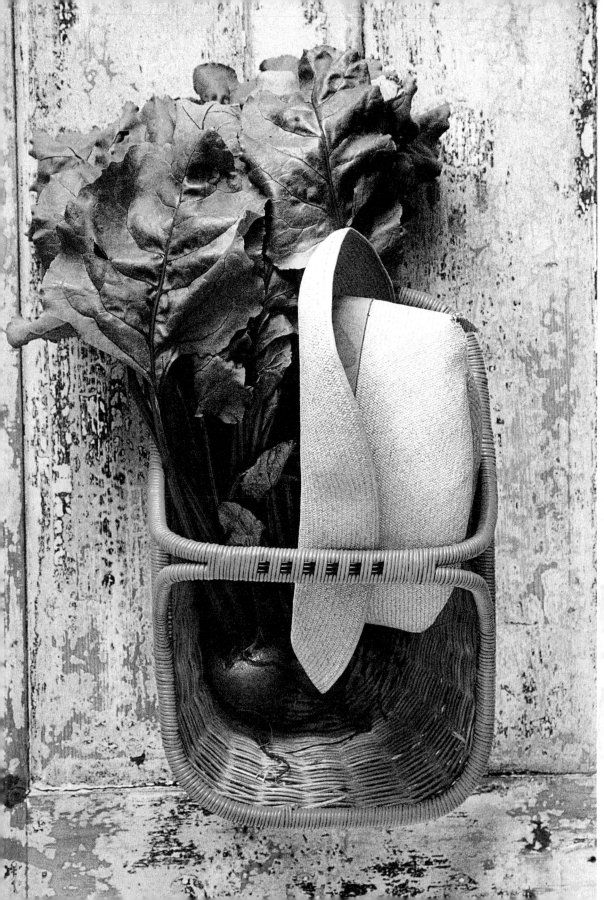

from season
to season

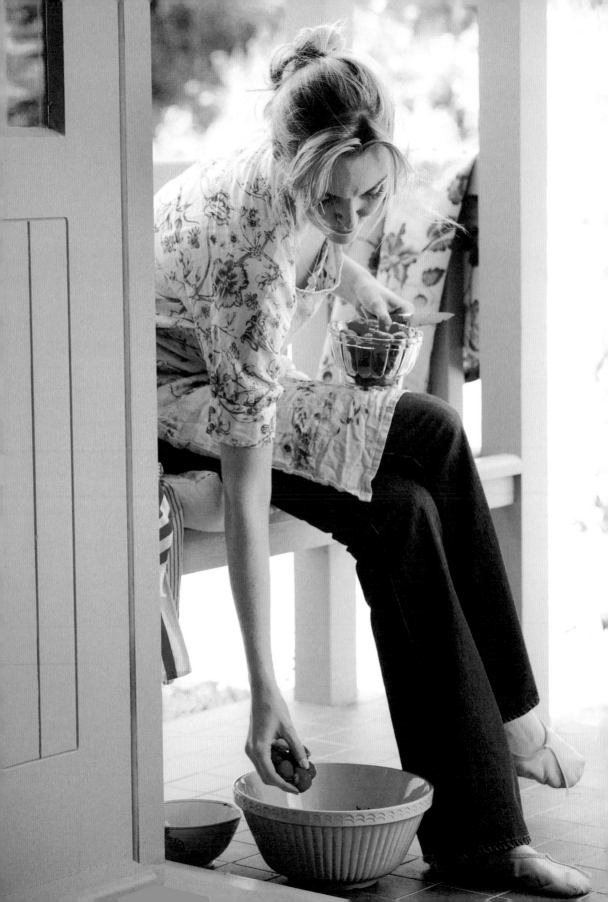

from season to season
a year in recipes
by Sophie Dahl

photographs by Jan Baldwin

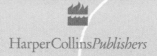

HarperCollins*Publishers*

For my Jamie, as everything is.

And to my grandmother, Patsy Louise, who had
the courage of a lion and loved her family, along
with avocados, cheap wine and hymns.

SD

HarperCollins*Publishers*
77–85 Fulham Palace Road,
Hammersmith, London W6 8JB

www.harpercollins.co.uk

First published by HarperCollins in 2011

10 9 8 7 6 5 4 3 2 1

Image on pg111 © getty images

A catalogue record of this book is
available from the British Library

ISBN 978-0-00-734051-4

Printed and bound in the UK by
Butler Tanner & Dennis Ltd, Frome, Somerset

Art Director: Patrick Budge
Photographer: Jan Baldwin
Food Stylist: Alice Hart
Props Stylist: Emma Thomas

Contents

Cook's notes

All pepper is freshly ground black pepper. I also like to use a coarse sea salt like Maldon.

I'm a big believer in free-range, cruelty-free produce. To that end, try and buy dairy and meat from a supplier you trust, one who treats their animals with respect.

We are overfishing our painfully understocked oceans. To get a list of what fish are sustainable and plentiful, please go to the Marine Stewardship Council website (the MSC) www.msc.org.

Stock: I use fresh or, if being lazy, Marigold Vegetable Bouillon or Kallo's Organic Free-range Chicken Stock.

Good usefuls to have in the larder and fridge, in no particular order and given in haphazard fashion:

Belazu Balsamic Vinegar (really
 thick and syrupy)
Miso paste (for dressings and
 marinades)
Rice vinegar
Tahini
Pomegranate molasses
A good, strong mustard
Tamari
Mirin
Marsala
Horseradish root
A bunch of fresh herbs
 Tarragon
 Parsley
 Coriander
 Chives
Argan oil
Pumpkin seed oil
Some good-quality dark
chocolate
Some cheap chocolate for eating
 on the spur of the moment or
 when miserable

Lemons for zesting
Chickpeas
Lentils (both Puy and yellow)
A good home-made garam
 masala
Star anise
Cardamom
Arborio rice
An onion
Some garlic
Pearl barley for soups and stews
Arrowroot for thickening gravies
 or sauces for the gluten-free
Spelt flour
Good vanilla extract
Runny honey
Fresh coffee
Stock in ice-cube trays in the
 freezer
Sunflower seeds to toast and
 add to salads and bread

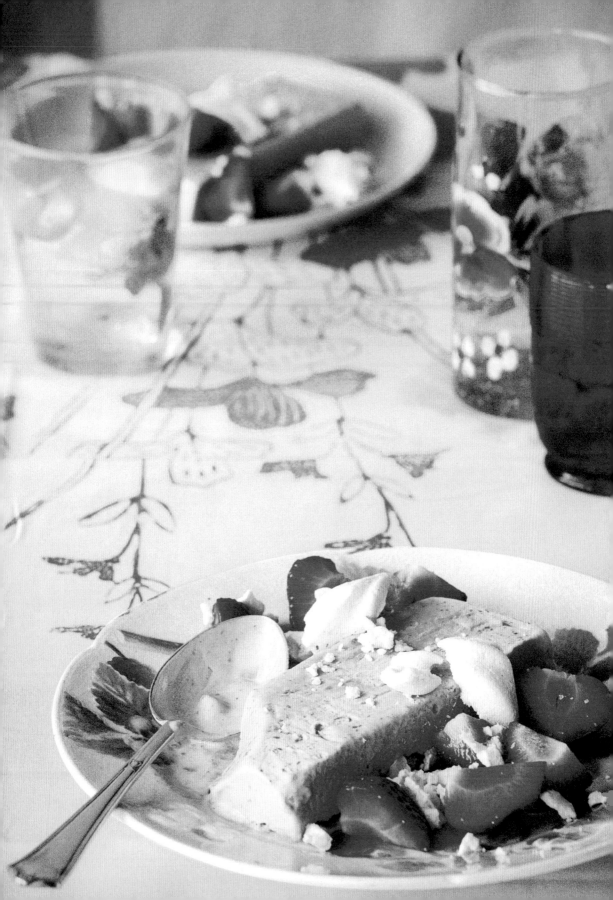

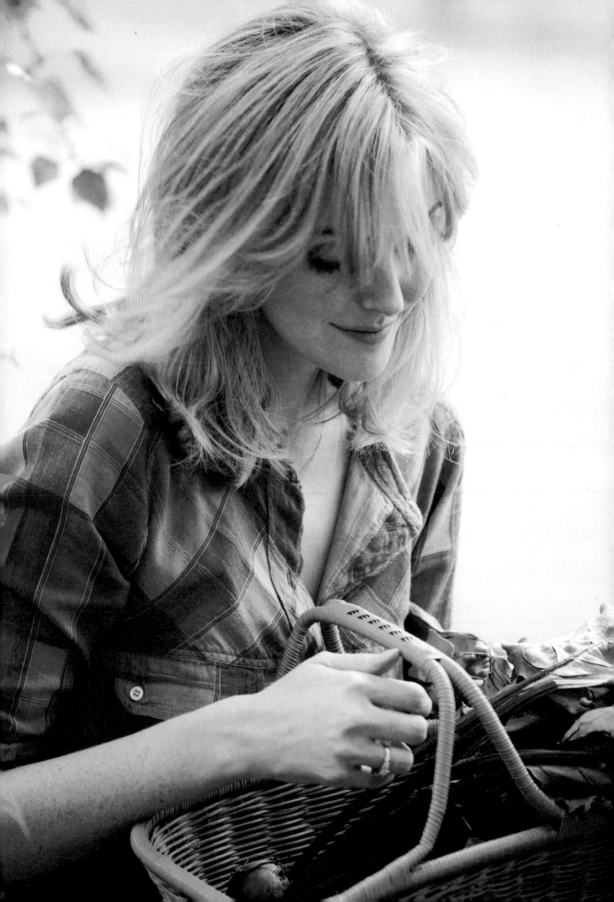

Introduction

'It's a question of discipline,' The Little Prince told me later on. 'When you've finished washing and dressing each morning, you must tend to your planet.'
Antoine de Saint-Exupéry, *The Little Prince*

In my last book, *Miss Dahl's Voluptuous Delights*, I began with writing that many of our grandparents ate healthfully and seasonally before there was a name for it, eating with an innate common sense and practicality that somehow, along the way, many of us have forgotten. This doesn't stand for everyone's grandparents, as I discovered on a book tour to Denmark. A journalist there asked me if I knew what her grandparents were eating fifty years ago. I knew from her smile I was on treacherous ground and took a deep breath of preparation.

'No,' I demurred politely. 'What did they eat?'

'LARD!' She said. 'They lived on lard and potatoes! I eat far better than they would have ever dreamed! What do you think of that Miss home-grown-seasonal-vegetable-garden-have-a-walk-every-day?'

I immediately morphed into a filmic parody of Hugh Grant and said something very English and vague like, 'Well, yes, I don't know what everyone's grandparents ate, hmm, easy to generalize, mutter, ho hum.' And blushed.

Under the gaze of watchful Danes, I stand corrected then, and speak only for my own grandparents, who grew fruit and vegetables in their garden, buying fish from the local fishmonger, meat from the local butcher and dairy from their local farmer. Every meal on their table came to fruition with an unspoken nod to seasonality and availability.

I am keenly aware that if you are a busy working parent, or if you live somewhere isolated, sometimes all that is on offer (or is bearable) is a one-stop shop. I am sometimes guilty of it myself. But I also believe that if each one of us makes a concession towards being a conscious consumer, we are in turn making an active contribution to looking after our lovely planet, which has enough exterior torment going on in it without us adding to it.

We are blessed in England to have our very definite seasons. Sometimes they feel never ending, dragging winter in particular, but the reward is tangible, both in the garden and on the plate. There is a finite certainty to the seasons that I, as a neurotic ever pursuer of order, find blissfully predictable.

I like knowing that on a damp autumn evening, whilst the wind is pounding at the windows, I can transport myself with a bowl of molten comfort, a soup of squash and Parmesan, served with a thick hunk of buttered bread. This is when food meets the call of the weather, as it's hard to imagine the summer when it's been replaced by lashing rain. The memory of a ceviche, tart with lime, can propel you through the darkest days of winter, carrying you right to the moment when you can actually eat it in the garden, as drowsy bees sail past, the air throbbing with sun and lavender.

I come from a long tradition of home cooks. I write about some of them here. England is full of them, hundreds upon thousands of them practically more skilled than I. You only have to look within one of the many branches of the Women's Institute or similar to find women whose lemon bars are like the tender tears of an angel, whose puff pastry flakes with an unparalleled buttery grace. I worship at the altar of these culinary high priestesses. I still can't chop an onion properly, and my apple coring looks like the prelude to a horror film. I very occasionally make a cake that could be used as a weapon or forget to put the sugar in something. I am content with this haphazard state of affairs; it keeps me honest. I own an apple corer, and I make whoever is lurking in the kitchen around Sunday lunch time chop my onions. I lob shards of my occasional missile cakes at the voracious crows poaching my raspberries. I happen to be a greedy writer who likes to cook and then write about what I've cooked, not a chef, or a teacher. If you are looking for a voice of stern culinary authority, go elsewhere! I can give you stories, and ideas for things, along with food that is lovely, simple and straightforward. No forgotten sugar either, I promise. This book is a collection of recipes that were either written down as they were cooked, imagined late one sleepless night and then realized, admired and reprinted, or passed down by a stoic Norwegian great grandmother. They are all pretty easy, with minimal fussing required. I like honest cooking that speaks for itself, cooking that begs for seconds and a satisfied smile, and I truly hope that resonates from my kitchen to yours.

In the in-between, I wish for you an army of onion choppers, sponge that is light as a feather, soufflés that defy gravity and, if all else fails, a shoulder to cry on. Cooking is not tight-lipped and mean, and it is not judgmental either. It shouldn't be, and nor should eating. Both in their very nature are providers – of nourishment, family, warmth and community, alchemy and adventure.

So whether your grandparents were lard-eating Danes, Burmese farmers, molasses-eating Mississippians, prairie-sowing Middle Americans or, like mine, a mix of staunch Scandinavian, Scottish Presbyterian, Tennessee hillbillies and vegetable growing East Enders, most of all, I wish you happy eating. Whatever the season.

With love,

Sophie Dahl

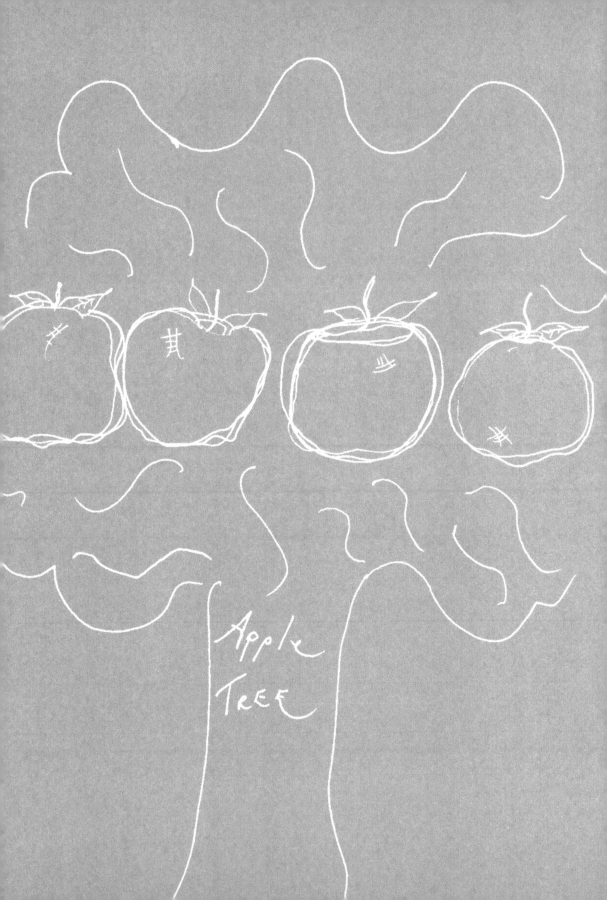

Autumn

BREAKFASTS
Tapioca with stewed apples and apricots
Argan oil, almond and honey smoothie
Crab cakes with poached eggs and spinach
Spelt French toast with smashed blueberries and blackberries
Mushrooms on toast
Apple cider omelette
Gooseberry yoghurt

LUNCHES
Heartbreak carbonara (or the first thing I ever cooked for a boy)
Squash and Parmesan soup
Spanish omelette
Baked pumpkin with lemon, sautéed greens and toasted
  cumin dressing
Soba noodle salad with rainbow vegetables and sesame dressing
Lentil salad with a mustard dressing
Beef Stroganoff

SUPPERS
Salmon steaks with a wasabi coating
Baked vegetables smothered in scamorza
Root vegetable cakes with a cheesy béchamel sauce
Tofu lasagne
Chickpea/garbanzo bean mushroom burgers with tahini sauce
Lentil pie
The first Mor Mor and her chicken

Autumn is all about nostalgia. For me it will forever be the season of back to school, first loves, and bonfire night. The food of autumn captures all of that in a net. Even the scent of autumn is sweet, smoky and wistful.

From four to seventeen I attended quite a few schools, from the call your teacher Bob and do yoga as a sport sort, to the white gloves and curtsying to the headmistress after prayers, draconian institute that is particular to England. The one constant in the merry-go-round was the familiar feeling that flooded to the surface during the last week of August, the week before the autumn term began. It was a cross between an itch and a promise, as the evenings grew colder and supper was suddenly hot soup or a baked potato. It was furthered by buying tights and the accoutrements of junior academia: shiny pencil cases, as yet unmarred with the initials of the boy who we all had a crush on, scratched on with a compass, and virginal geometry books, so hopeful without the vivid red crosses that were sure to come.

If it was boarding school, which it was for a bit, there was the heart-plunging goodbye at the train station on a Sunday evening, the inevitable pall of rain steaming up the windows, staining the summer with a tearful goodbye. At day school, the first-day rain ceased to be a symbolic backdrop for all that was ill in the world, and more of a vanity irritant, mussing up the fringe that was so carefully straightened the night before, in honour of the sixth form boys.

Your classmates felt new like pennies, and you saw them with new eyes, at least for a day or two. Chloe now had a chest to rival Jane Russell; Joe's voice had broken and he had freckles from some faraway sun. Lola had a worldly weariness that could have something to do with a Greek waiter, and fat Robert was now thin and mean with it. Our teachers struggled with the new us, trying to gauge our emotional temperature with the old jokes that used to work, before we went and grew quietly behind their backs. So much can happen in ten weeks. Long gone from school, I still know that much can shift in a summer.

Maybe this is why autumn makes me so nostalgic. The tangible chrysalis effect of what's changed. I watch it now with my younger cousins and the children of friends. Fun fairs and post graduation nights of camping in places that parents would balk at, sangria and sunburn, and thinking you're in love with a person who can barely say hello in your language. Discovering that some friends won't, as you thought, walk into adult life with you, that all of those nights spent whispering secrets when the lights were out will be instead relegated to the yellowing pages of a diary.

During the summer I was in Los Angeles, far, far away from the thought of rain, tights or cosy autumnal food. I stayed at my aunt's house, which was filled with kids home from college for the summer and her menagerie of animals, including a bowl of violently coloured jellyfish and Frances Bacon, her pot-bellied pig. Frances is of variable temper, enormous and partially blind, she hates babies and cats in no particular order. She is very fond of strawberries, bed and sitting on the dogs, who live in mortal fear of her. We have always got on reasonably well. This all changed when my aunt went away for a week. Although I did all the things Frances likes – scratching her ears, rubbing sunscreen on her broad scaly back, feeding her banana skins and tucking her in at night – I think she connected my arrival with my aunt's disappearance and decided, like an errant stepchild, to make my life complicated. She crept stealthily into the larder (my favourite place) and trapped me there daily, blocking my exit with her two hundred pound bulk, trying to bite me if I attempted to get past her. We engaged in a ridiculous game that involved me holding a spoonful of strawberries aloft, and dancing from the kitchen into the garden like a pig Pied Piper, depositing the fruit into her open milky mouth, and running as fast as I could to lock the door behind me to the sound of porcine fury. In defeated distress, I called my aunt's assistant Sharon and explained the situation.

'Here's the thing,' she said, in dulcet Zen tones. I took a deep breath and wondered what Doctor Dolittle trick she was going to impart, 'It's very simple. Frances doesn't like change.'

In the spirit of change, I give you the following. It's for leaf-sodden days and misty mornings.

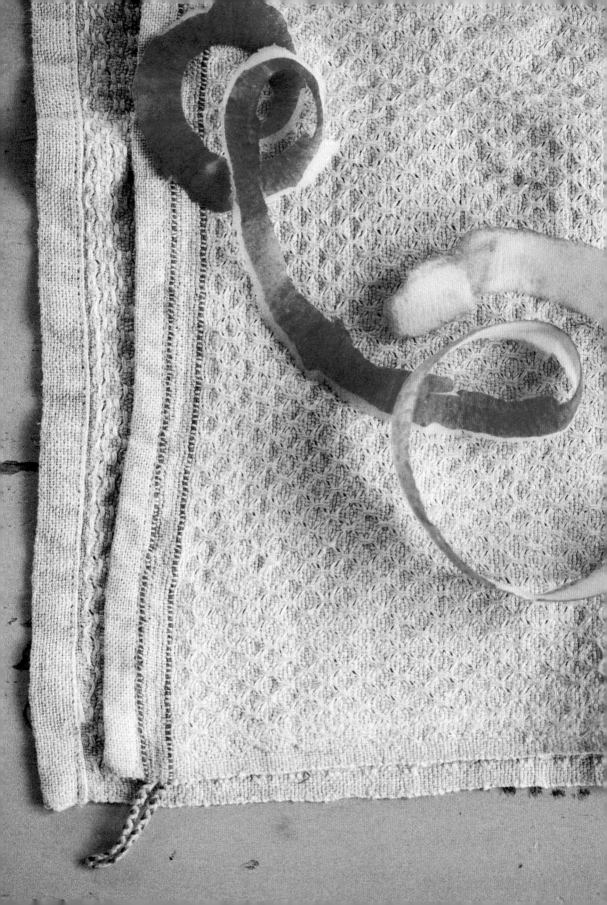

Autumn
Breakfasts

Tapioca with stewed apples and apricots

Tapioca, like semolina, is one of those things that a school kitchen could have turned you off for life. I couldn't eat it for years, having been force-fed it at primary school aged six, with tinned jam, as it oozed like frogspawn out of the bowl, and I wept and retched. For years I had the same malicious feeling towards beetroot and mashed potatoes, which were instant and came in lumpy granules. My teacher and I had a silent war every lunch time; a war that eventually came to an end after my parents removed me from the school. Made to your own wont, in your own kitchen, tapioca is ambrosial, and worth being a grown-up for, as is semolina. This could also be a pudding not a breakfast, just don't serve it with dog food-like tinned jam. Try a lovely home-made compote instead.

Having soaked the tapioca overnight, drain and place it in a saucepan with the milk, vanilla extract and a knob of butter. Bring to the boil, turn to low and simmer, stirring in the honey, agave or sugar, for another 10 minutes.

Cut your overnight magically plumped apricots into halves or quarters if desired. In another saucepan, place the water, cinnamon, orange juice, agave or honey and apple and bring to the boil, giving it a good stir now and then. Simmer for about 10 to 15 minutes or until the apple is tender.

Now, here you can do one of two things. Serve the stewed fruit as is on top of the tapioca or put the tapioca in a small ovenproof dish with another knob of butter, pour the apple and apricot on top and bake at 180°C/160°C fan/Gas 4 for 15 or so minutes. The choice, Cilla, is yours.

SERVES 4

70g/½ cup of tapioca (soaked overnight in plenty of water)

350ml/1⅓ cups of milk

1 teaspoon of vanilla extract

A knob of butter

2 tablespoons of runny honey or agave syrup or brown sugar

For the apple and apricots

12 dried apricots (like the tapioca, soaked overnight, but in about 250ml/1 cup of orange juice)

250ml/1 cup or so of water

1 cinnamon stick

A few tablespoons of orange juice

1 tablespoon of agave syrup or honey

2 eating apples, peeled, cored and sliced

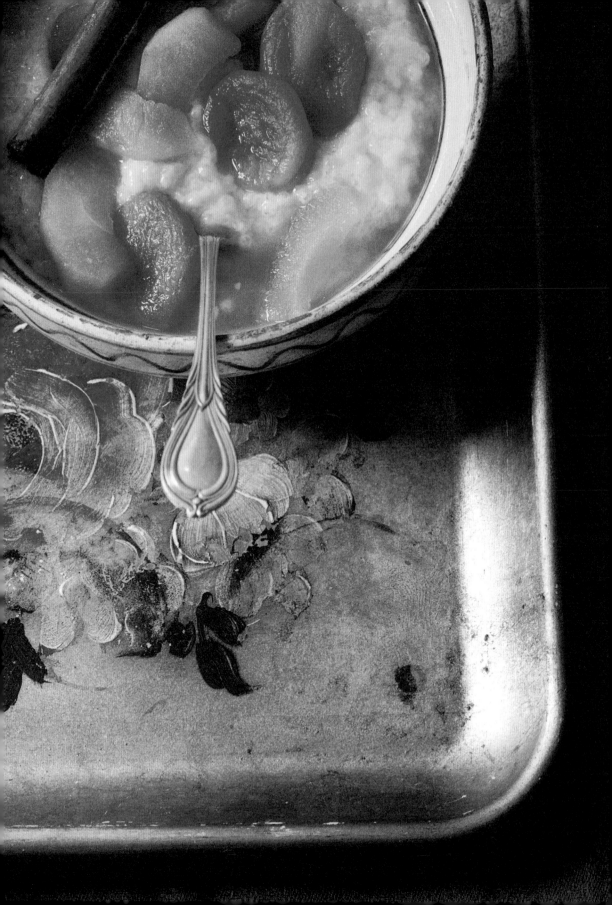

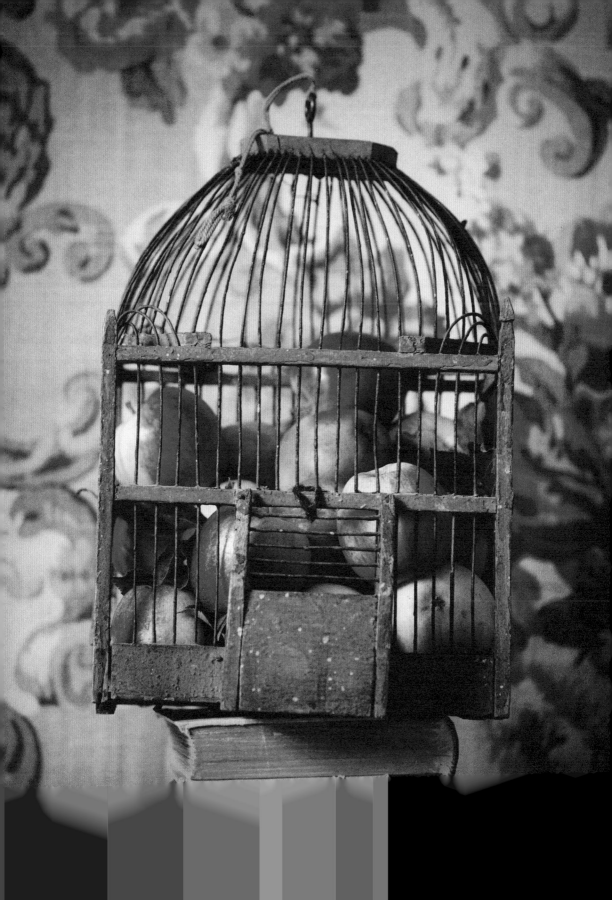

Argan oil, almond and honey smoothie

SERVES 1

½ a frozen banana
8 or so blanched almonds
1 glass of soy milk
1 teaspoon of Argan oil
1 tablespoon of runny
  honey

Argan oil comes from the Argan tree, a Moroccan tree with magical properties. The oil is now easy to obtain through mail order or online, or if you live in a city, at your local health food shop. I get mine from Wild Wood Groves, www.wildwoodgroves.com. If you can't access it, use a cold-pressed oil instead, something like an almond oil. I eat Argan, put it on my face and in my bath. It's also great for babies with eczema. Frozen bananas are perfect for adding to smoothies, so have some in stock. Chop up the banana and put it in the freezer in a Ziploc bag or Tupperware.

Put your banana, almonds, soy and Argan in the blender with your honey. Blend until smooth and drink and be joyful.

Crab cakes with poached eggs and spinach

Perhaps the thing I miss most about living in the US is the ubiquity of brunch, or the ready availability of breakfast foods in a restaurant, long after breakfast is normally finished. Crab cakes are such a thing, perfectly so with eggs on top. If the mountain can't come to Mohammed…

Get the crab cake mixture ready, by mixing all the ingredients, bar the egg and olive oil, and forming into little cakes. Beat the egg and brush the crab cakes with it, then heat the olive oil in a non-stick pan. Throw on the crab cakes and cook them for a few minutes on each side until golden. You can also wilt the spinach in the same pan for a few minutes. Plate, with the spinach around the crab cakes.

In another pan, boil some water with a dash of vinegar and some salt. When it is simmering away, carefully add your eggs and poach for 3 minutes. Drain and put the eggs on top of the crab cakes. Eat immediately.

SERVES 2

For the crab cakes
450g/1lb of cooked crab meat – white and brown
1 tablespoon of home-made or good mayonnaise
1 teaspoon of mustard
A few drops of Tabasco sauce
A small handful of fresh mixed herbs – dill, chervil and parsley
Salt and pepper
1 egg
2 tablespoons of olive oil

A handful of spinach
A dash of vinegar
Salt
2 eggs

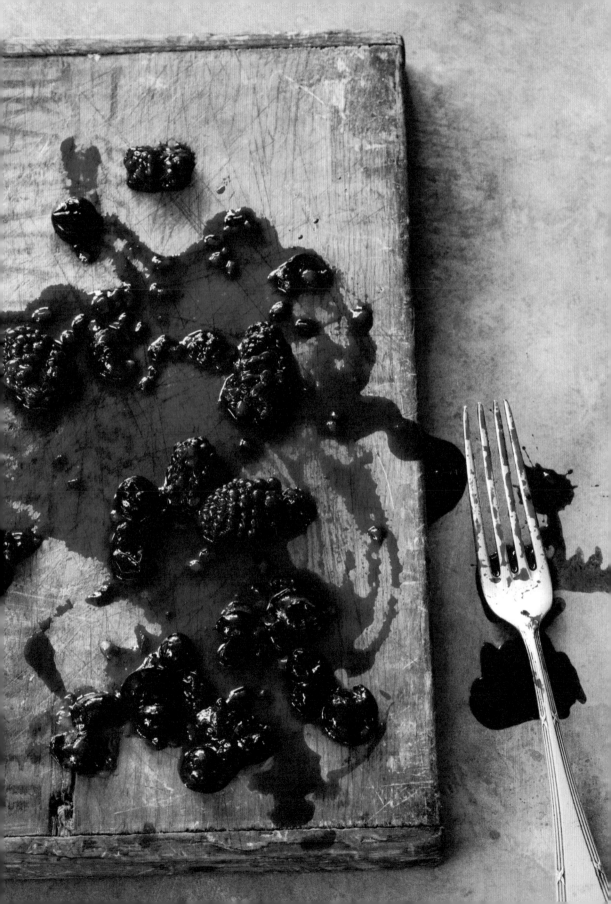

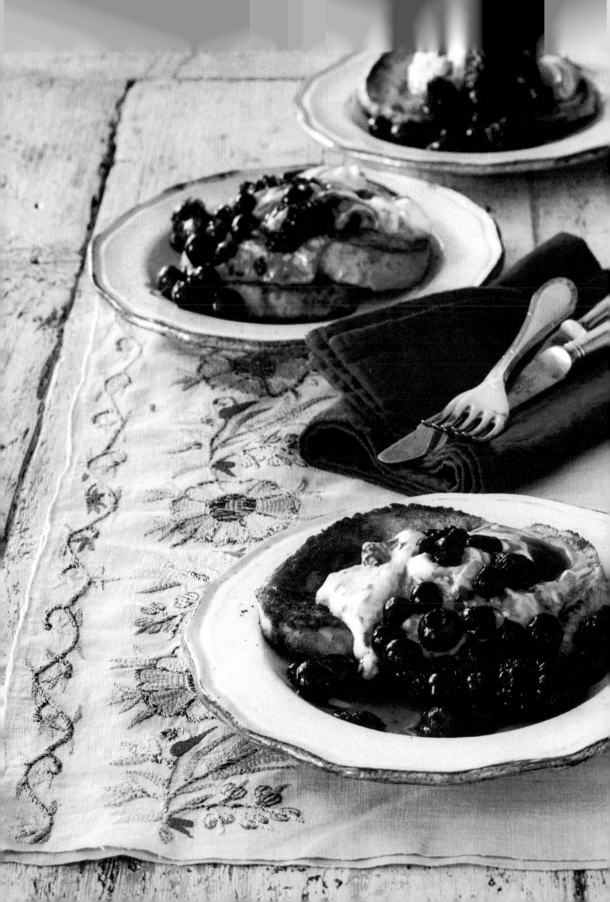

Spelt French toast with smashed blueberries and blackberries

SERVES 4

A day-old spelt loaf

4 eggs, plus 1 egg yolk

125ml/½ cup of milk

1 teaspoon of vanilla
   extract

2 tablespoons of agave
   syrup or brown sugar

Pinch of salt

1 tablespoon of butter

For the smashed
blueberries and
blackberries

2 generous handfuls each
   of blackberries and
   blueberries

1 tablespoon of water

3 tablespoons of agave
   syrup or honey

4 heaped tablespoons of
   Greek yoghurt

Another very happy childhood food memory. French toast is as comforting as a feather-filled bed.

Put the berries in a saucepan with the water and agave or honey. Bring to the boil and simmer for a few minutes, or until they begin to split into a big jammy autumnal mess.

Slice the stale loaf into manageable toast-sized pieces. In a mixing bowl, beat together the eggs and egg yolk with the milk, vanilla, agave or sugar and the pinch of salt. When well incorporated, pour this mixture into a shallow baking dish. Start putting the bread in it, making sure it's fully dunked. You need to let the bread sit in this eggy bath for at least 20 minutes, so it can really soak it up. If the bread needs help, prick it with a fork to help the egg mixture permeate.

Take a big griddle pan or large heavy-bottomed frying pan and melt the butter. Put the egg-soaked bread in, in batches if needs be. Cook it for about 4 minutes on each side, until the bread is bronzed on the outside and soft on the in. Serve on warmed plates, with the smashed berries and yoghurt on top.

Mushrooms on toast

This is also perfect for a Sunday night supper when there are few around and you can eat this on your lap, a poached egg on top of it, watching a good old costume drama.

First of all, make sure your pan is searing hot. Otherwise, your mushrooms can get soggy and unpleasant and, frankly, a soggy mushroom is a bit grim. Toss in the mushrooms at the same time as the olive oil and the garlic. You should hear an angry hiss. Hurrah!

Keep throwing it all around and when the mushrooms are the burnished shade that appeals to you, toss in the parsley, tarragon and butter. There should be lots of juices in the pan and I suggest you add to them with a trickle of cream. And maybe a splash of white wine? But I suppose it is breakfast. Season to taste and serve on crispy buttered toast with a big cup of tea.

SERVES 2

A good few handfuls of mixed wild mushrooms, roughly chopped

1 tablespoon of olive oil

1 clove of garlic, peeled and finely chopped

A handful of fresh parsley

A pinch of fresh chopped tarragon

A knob of butter

A whisper of single/light cream

Salt and pepper

Slices of soda bread or dark rye, toasted and buttered

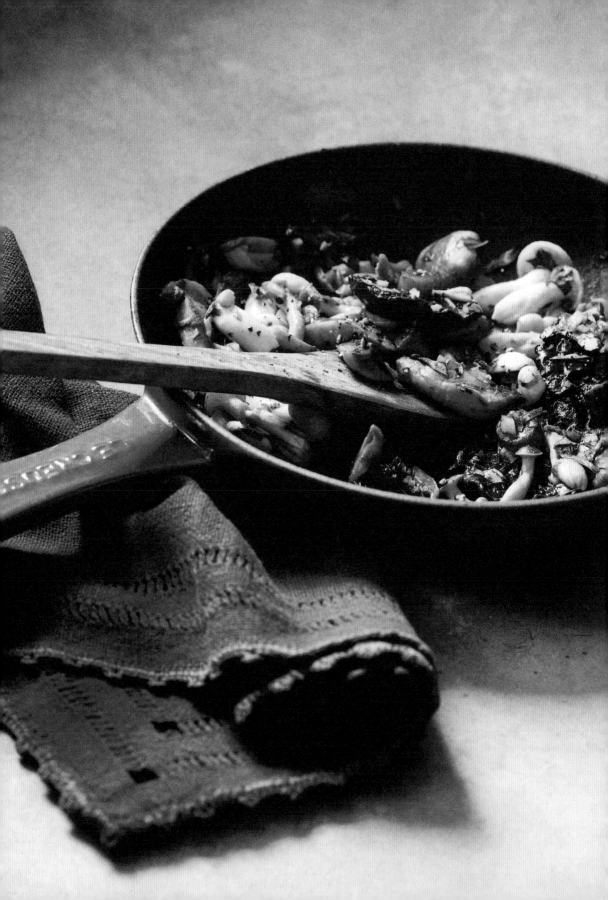

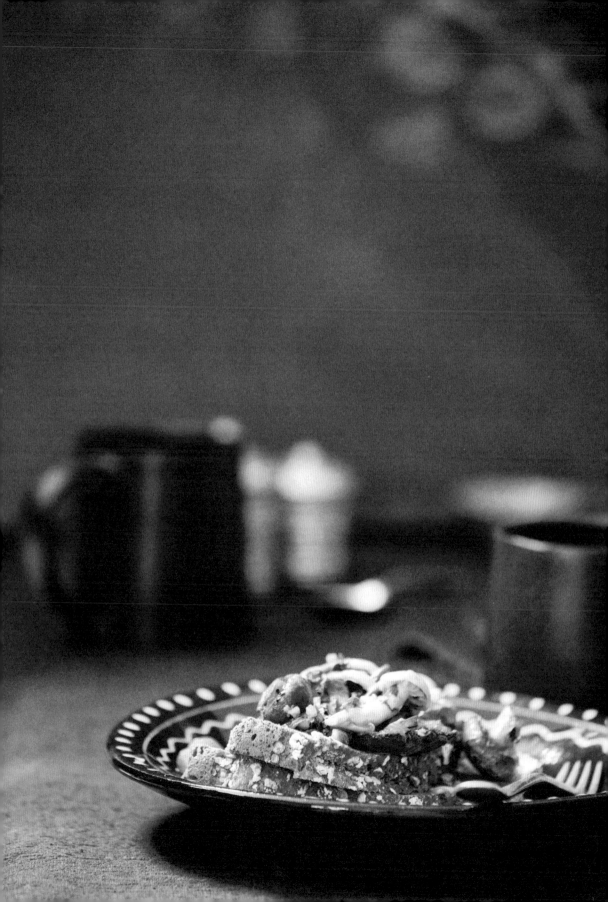

Apple cider omelette

SERVES 1

2 tablespoons of butter

¼ of a small onion, peeled and finely chopped

2 teaspoons of apple cider vinegar

Salt and pepper

3 eggs

50g/½ cup of mature/sharp Cheddar cheese, grated

1 teaspoon of sumac

1 teaspoon of fresh chopped thyme

There is nothing more English nor more autumnal than an apple swollen from the tree in late September. This omelette celebrates that in my house. Put your scarf on and kick some leaves!

Melt 1 tablespoon of butter, on a medium heat, in a non-stick frying pan. Add the onion and turn the heat down, cooking until it is soft. Add the apple cider vinegar and season, cooking until the vinegar is absorbed. Whisk the eggs and, adding the rest of the butter to the frying pan, pour in the eggs over the onion mixture, making sure it's distributed easily. Agitate it a bit and add the Cheddar, sumac and thyme. Flip it, cooking for another 30 seconds or so until cooked, and serve.

Gooseberry yoghurt

Dedicated to my Aunt Lucy – a gooseberry fan. So much so that when she was in Amsterdam and saw gooseberries on the menu, she began shouting 'Gooseberries!' at the top of her voice and did a little joyous dance, much to the amusement of my cousins, her daughters. She does live in Los Angeles, so is gooseberry deprived, rather than just a bit weird.

Preheat the oven to 180°C/160°C fan/Gas 4. Put the gooseberries in an ovenproof baking dish and sprinkle with the sugar and orange flower water. Cook, uncovered, for about 20 minutes, take out and leave to cool thoroughly. Strain the gooseberries, pour into the blender and purée for a minute or so.

This can be eaten in a multitude of ways. Pour on the top of the yoghurt so it drips through, leave on the bottom of the yoghurt to find as a surprise or ribbon through it.

SERVES 4

400g/14oz of gooseberries

2 tablespoons of brown sugar

1 teaspoon of orange flower water

185ml/¾ cup of Greek yoghurt

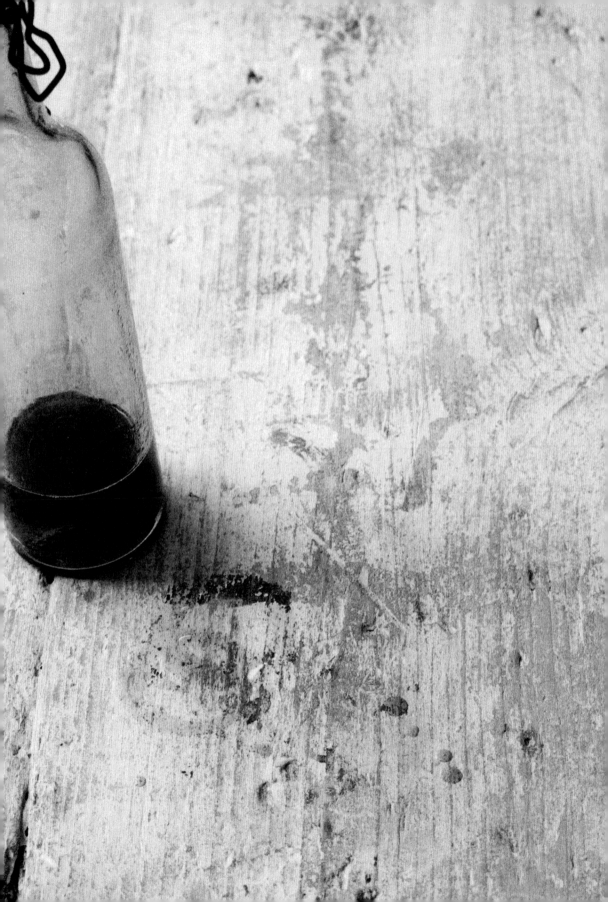

Autumn
Lunches

Heartbreak carbonara (or the first thing I ever cooked for a boy)

SERVES 4

125g/4½ oz of pancetta, bacon or ham
2 tablespoons of olive oil
4 egg yolks
30g/¼ cup of grated Parmesan
A splash of white wine
2 tablespoons of single/light cream
Salt and pepper
500g/1lb 2oz of spaghetti

To marry with the wistful theme of my autumn, here is the first thing I ever cooked for a boy who I loved quietly and secretly. The carbonara in the pan lingered longer than he did — he wolfed it down with a bottle of Chianti, and informed me he was actually in love with a dancer called Willow (or something infinitely more exotic than Sophie). Then he disappeared into the night. I lay sobbing on the floor, wishing I could be angular and coordinated like Willow. Indeed, I cried such a ridiculous amount that in the morning I looked as if I had a black eye, and my mother gave me a heartbreak dispensation day off school.

Cut the pancetta into bite-sized pieces. In a medium-sized frying pan, put a small glug of oil and cook the pancetta until crispy. Put to the side.

In a mixing bowl, beat together the egg yolks, Parmesan, splash of wine, the cream and some salt and pepper. Add the pancetta and mix it all together. Cook the pasta and, as soon as it is ready, mix it quickly with the sauce so the egg doesn't cook.

Heartbreak not essential.

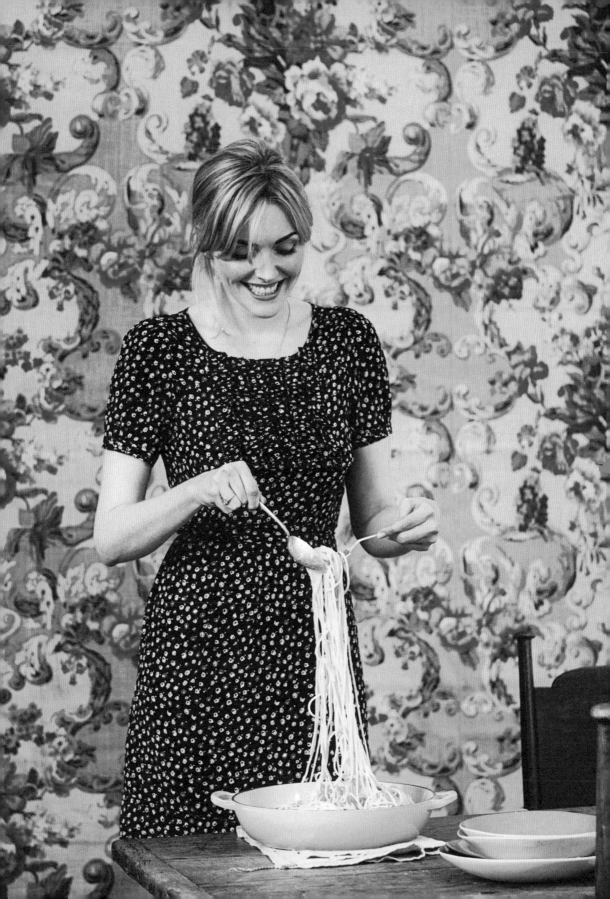

Squash and Parmesan soup

SERVES 4

50g/½ stick of butter

1kg/2lb of squash, cubed

1 onion, peeled and finely
chopped

1 clove of garlic, peeled and
finely chopped

2 tablespoons of sherry

875ml/3½ cups of chicken
or vegetable stock

½ teaspoon of cayenne
pepper

A couple of bay leaves

Salt and pepper

2 tablespoons of
double/heavy cream

A handful of toasted
pumpkin seeds

A handful of fresh
chopped parsley

A handful of grated
Parmesan

This is what blowsy October days are made for. Comforting and golden, this soup is a hymn to autumn. I first made this clucking around in upstate New York when I had some leftover squash. It works just as well with pumpkin or sweet potato.

In a heavy-bottomed pan, melt the butter and add the squash, onion and garlic. Cook for a few minutes. Add the sherry, stir and then add the stock, cayenne pepper and bay leaves. Cook until the squash is tender, about 10 to 15 minutes. Remove the bay leaves and blend the soup either with a hand-held mixer or in the blender. Season and add the cream. Serve with a topping of pumpkin seeds, parsley and grated Parmesan.

Spanish omelette

Like a frittata, a bit of a recycling dish for what you've got lying around. Also great for a lunchbox for a small or big person – just wrap in greaseproof/wax paper.

Preheat the grill to a high setting. In a large non-stick frying pan, heat 2 tablespoons of the oil on a medium to low flame. Add the potatoes and the onions and cook until golden. Take off the heat and reserve.

Whisk the eggs and season them. Pour the onion and potato mixture into the eggs and heat another tablespoon of olive oil in the pan. Add the egg, potato and onion and turn the heat down to low. Loosen the edges and agitate the pan.

When the bottom is set and golden brown, take an oiled plate, turn the omelette out and put it back in the pan, this time face-side down. Transfer the omelette to under a hot grill and cook for another minute or two until the top is set, then turn out, serving happily either hot or cold.

SERVES 4

3 tablespoons of olive oil
225g/1½ cups of potatoes, peeled and thinly sliced
150g/1⅓ cups of onions, thinly sliced
8 eggs
Salt and pepper

Bonfire night

I had been raiding the memory bank in order to come up with a recipe that captured all of the hissing November glory of Bonfire Night, but I first arrived at a feeling rather than a taste. Whether wrapped in the crisp skin of a twice-baked potato, or hidden amidst the charred sweetness of a sausage, rolling anticipation is the abiding sense of that night for me. Maybe it's a hangover from those teenage days – crushes seen through a wreath of bonfire smoke, against a backdrop of technicoloured sky, or the electric feel of cold fingers handing over an oozing marshmallow. Either way, the visuals are made flesh as soon as you eat something with a November tinge, from jaw-locking candy apples to mellow roasted pumpkin, and how....

'Fireworks in the heavens, fireworks in my head, one vodka too many, now I wish I was dead.'

These were the words I wrote on the sixth of November, aged seventeen, nursing an aching head and heart. I had seen my love rat ex-boyfriend across a bonfire the night before and, oh woe, necked a couple of stiff vodkas and wobbled up to him, professing undying affection in the face of his horrible cheating ways. Love rat was a classic; twenty-seven to my seventeen, he'd disappear for nights on end and then eventually return with love bites and a bedraggled bouquet, probably nicked from a grave. He never had any money and was constantly dipping into my babysitting funds, and he only ever wore a black polo neck, probably to hide the love bites.

On that night of sparklers, over the smell of chestnuts, he greeted my tear thick protestations with fluttering eyelashes and a sly smile.

'Oh sweetheart, I've been away. Went to see a man about a dog in Leicester, you know how it is.'

I didn't know how it was – how could I? I was green as a milk-fed calf, and I thought that if I just looked after him, made him lasagne and kept him warm, he would love me as he had in August, and he might even stop drinking and disappearing. And after all, weren't the greatest love affairs meant to be a bit tortured in their onset? I was highly romantic and believed we were playing out a drama of old, I Caitlin to his Dylan, or he Burton to my Taylor.

As my friends rolled their eyes around the bonfire, he kissed me behind a bush, and then sloped home to his new girlfriend, a twenty-something Dane with stumpy legs, a BMW and her own flat in Chelsea. I did not have a flat in Chelsea; I lived in Balham with my mum, had a curfew and I couldn't drive.

'He doesn't really love her,' I told my friend Cassie afterwards, the relief of his kiss still reassuringly near. 'He loves me. He told me, it was very sincere. I feel awful for him. He feels beholden to the Dane because she doesn't know anyone in London, and he's painting her flat. It's temporary. And anyway, I have better legs.'

'Love,' she said. 'He's a total prat.'

'Aren't they all?' I asked wearily, as the Catherine wheels sang over my head. I felt that this was one of life's MOMENTS, one that I would remember always.

My association with the love rat lasted until Christmas, when the stumpy Dane who had stolen him from me called me crying. She read from my script, and I felt oddly sorry for her.

'He's gone missing,' she said.

'He does that,' I said. 'It's horrible.'

And as I said the things to her that everyone had said to me, it became real.

'You're worth more than this. Love is not meant to be about uncertainty. He's very lucky to have you.'

The truth was liberating.

'He's a total arse,' I told her. 'I'd get rid of him if I were you.'

It was November a good seven years later when I bumped into him. Red wine stained his teeth, and gathered in the creases of his mouth. He looked like a vampire and stumbled with drink. He told me I was the great love of his life. I laughed. He still wore a polo neck.

Baked pumpkin with lemon, sautéed greens and toasted cumin dressing

This is perfect to serve with some quinoa or wild rice as a main to a non-meat eater, or as a side with some roast chicken for the carnivorous. It's also good served warm the following day with a little grilled tofu added.

Preheat the oven to 220°C/200°C fan/Gas 7. Put the pumpkin in a roasting tray with the onion and sage, season, and pour over the olive oil. Cook for around 30 minutes or until the pumpkin is tender.

While the pumpkin is cooking, make your dressing. In a small frying pan on a medium heat, toast the cumin seeds. This should only take a minute, and you will know it's ready when the dusk of the cumin is wafting round your kitchen. Cool for a minute, then squeeze the lemon juice into the pan, followed by the olive oil. Put this into a jug or something and leave to the side, stirring the crème fraîche in just before serving.

Now, the greens. In a big frying pan, heat the olive oil and garlic. Throw in the greens and cook until tender, about 5 to 10 minutes.

Take the pumpkin out of the oven, put the greens on a plate, with the pumpkin on top and cover with the dressing.

SERVES 4

1kg/2lb of pumpkin, deseeded and chopped into rough chunks and/or slices
1 large red onion, peeled and roughly chopped
A few fresh sage leaves, roughly torn
Salt and pepper
2 tablespoons of olive oil

For the dressing
1½ teaspoons of cumin seeds or ground cumin
Juice of ½ a lemon
1 tablespoon of olive oil
1 teaspoon of crème fraîche/sour cream

For the sautéed greens
2 tablespoons of olive oil
1 clove of garlic, peeled and finely chopped
A handful of Swiss chard
A handful of curly kale

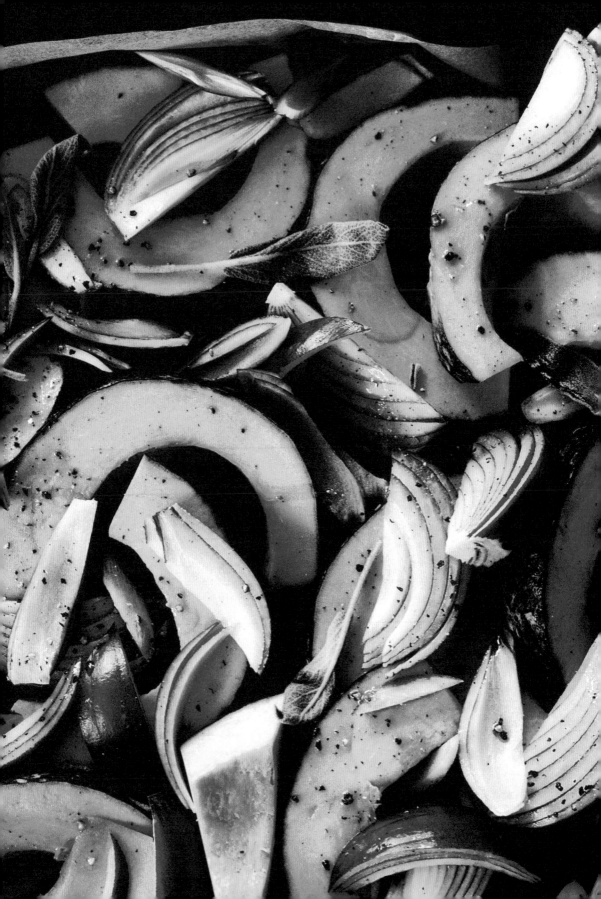

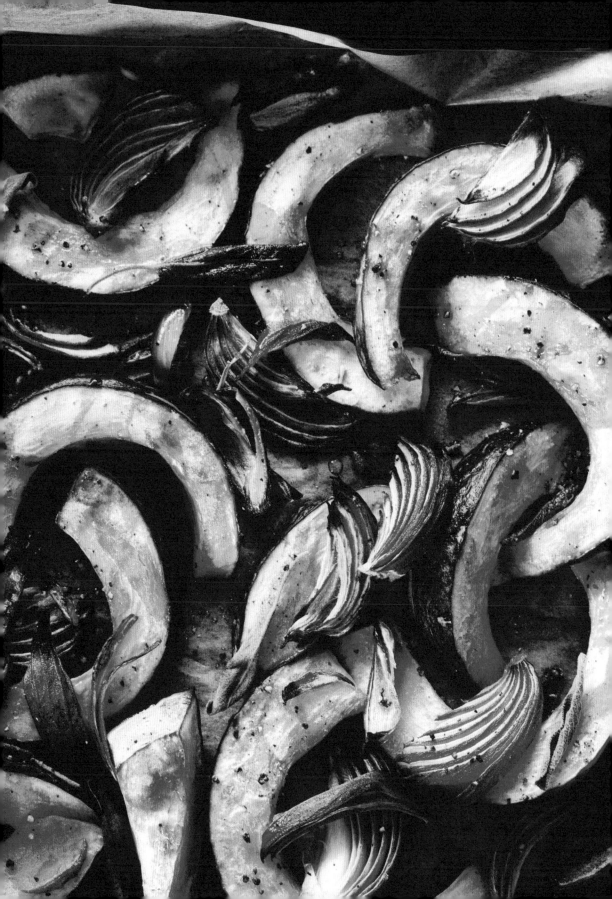

Soba noodle salad with rainbow vegetables and sesame dressing

SERVES 2

250g/9oz of soba noodles

⅓ of a large daikon (about 150g/5oz), cut into thin strips

½ a small head of white cabbage, shredded

1 medium carrot, grated

A handful of radishes, thinly sliced

1 spring onion/scallion, finely shredded

1 small handful of sesame seeds

For the dressing

3 tablespoons of sesame oil

1 tablespoon of brown rice vinegar

1 teaspoon of tamari (wheat-free soy sauce)

1 teaspoon of agave syrup or honey

I put soba noodles in everything – soups, salads and stir-fries. This is a quick, healthy, bountiful lunch and one to give to your friend who's allergic to EVERYTHING.

Cook the soba noodles by bringing 2 litres/8 cups of water to the boil, adding the noodles and cooking on low for 6 or so minutes. Drain and cool. When the noodles are cool, put them in the bowl you are planning to serve them in and add all of the vegetables – shredding, grating and thinly slicing.

In a small frying pan, toast the sesame seeds for a minute or so. Add to the noodles. Make the dressing by whisking all the ingredients together, adjusting according to taste, and pour over the noodles.

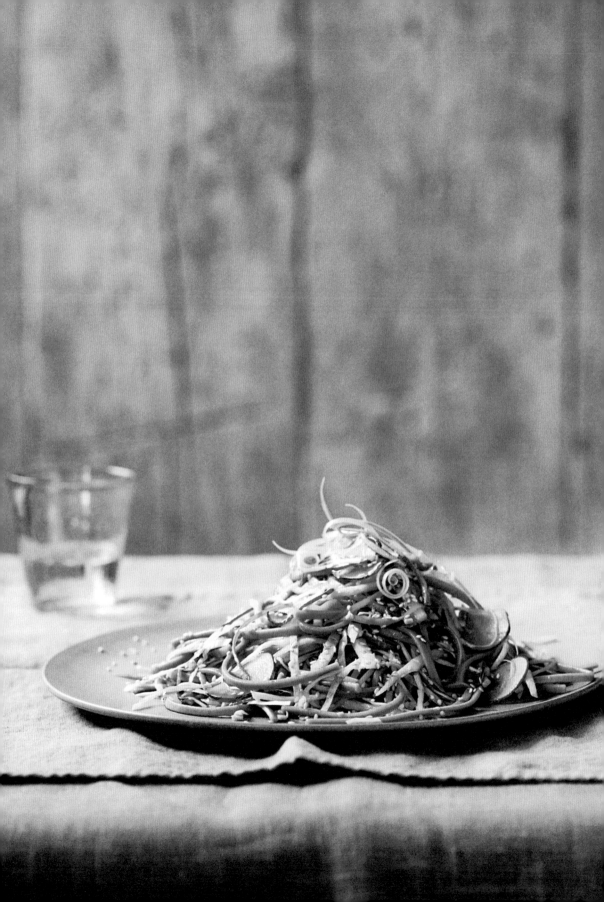

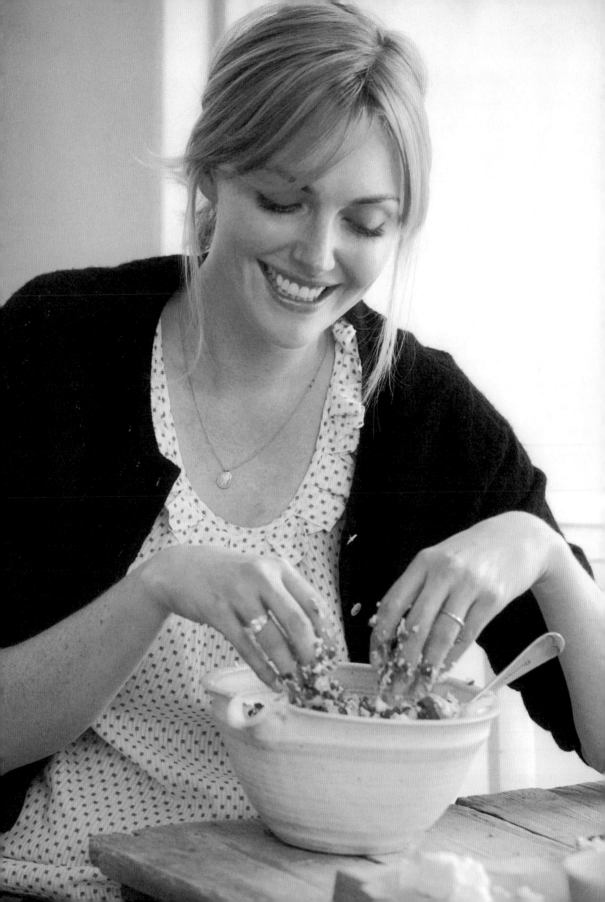

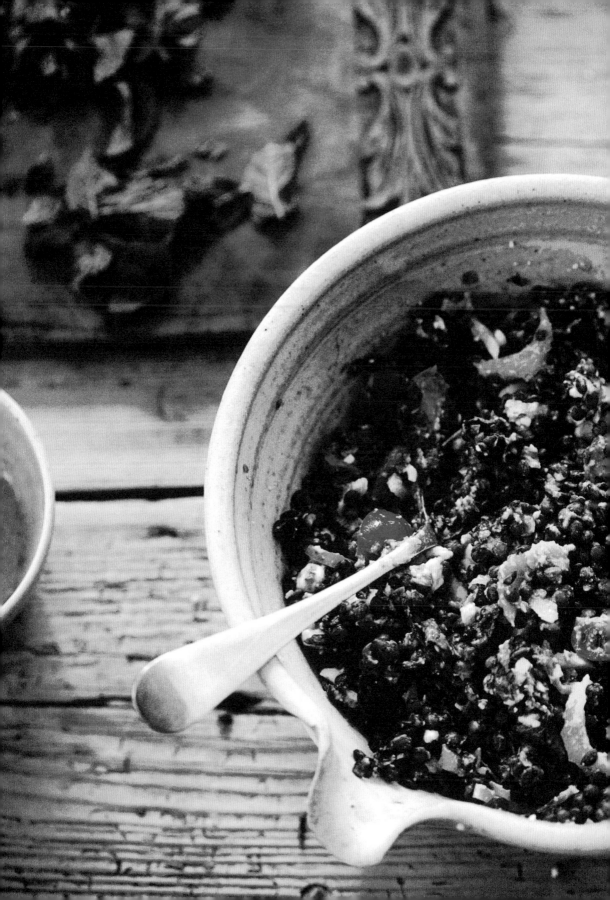

Lentil salad with a mustard dressing

SERVES 4

225g/1¼ cups of Puy lentils

2 celery sticks, chopped in fine rounds

A handful of cherry tomatoes, finely chopped

150g/1 cup of feta, crumbled

A small handful of fresh chopped mint

For the dressing

4 tablespoons of olive or rapeseed oil

1 teaspoon of white wine vinegar

2 teaspoons of Dijon mustard

1 shallot, peeled and finely chopped

Salt and pepper

Lentils are always good things to have in stock, along with chickpeas. You can turn them into a salad or soup on the spot. This is a hearty salad that is also good warm.

Place the lentils in a pan and add just enough water to cover. Simmer over a low heat for 20 minutes, then drain.

In a serving bowl, mix the lentils with the celery, tomatoes and feta.

Make the dressing by whisking all the ingredients together, adjusting according to taste. Dress the salad and then toss with the mint.

Beef Stroganoff

I know, I know. Totally from the same school as Chicken Kiev in terms of 80s nostalgia and naffness. But wasn't it good, particularly if it came in a ready meal? We knew not what we did. I used to beg for Beef Stroganoff as a child. I think, as a worthy vegetarian, it became Quorn Stroganoff and now, somewhere in the middle, the last time I had anything resembling it was a mushroom variety in a pub in Cornwall. Good old retro food.

Put a frying pan on a low heat and drop in the oil or butter. Add the onion and garlic and sweat for a few minutes, making sure they don't brown. Add the mushrooms and cook until they are golden. Put this mixture to the side.

In the same pan, heat a little more oil and add the beef strips, the paprika and the lemon. Toss around. Cook for a minute or so, and then splash on the vermouth. Pour the mushroom and onion mixture back in the pan, cook for another minute but no longer, and then take off the heat and add the sour cream and the parsley. Mix it all together and serve with some simple boiled potatoes or rice.

SERVES 4

1 tablespoon of olive oil or butter, plus extra oil

1 onion, peeled and finely chopped

1 clove of garlic, peeled and finely chopped

2 handfuls of mushrooms, roughly chopped

500g/1lb 2oz of beef fillet, chopped into strips 1cm/½ inch wide and thick

1 teaspoon of paprika

Juice of ½ a lemon

A splash of vermouth

60ml/¼ cup of sour cream

A handful of fresh chopped parsley

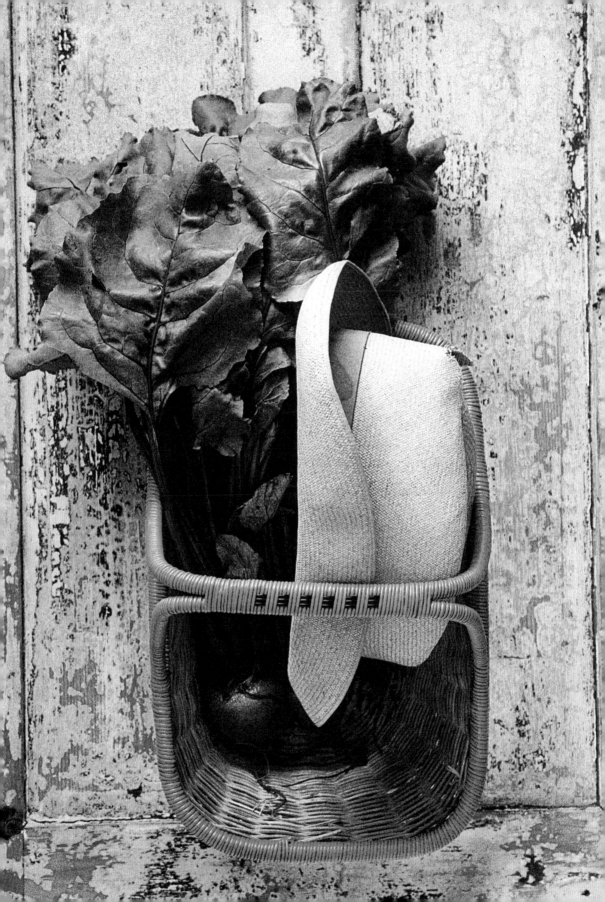

Autumn Suppers

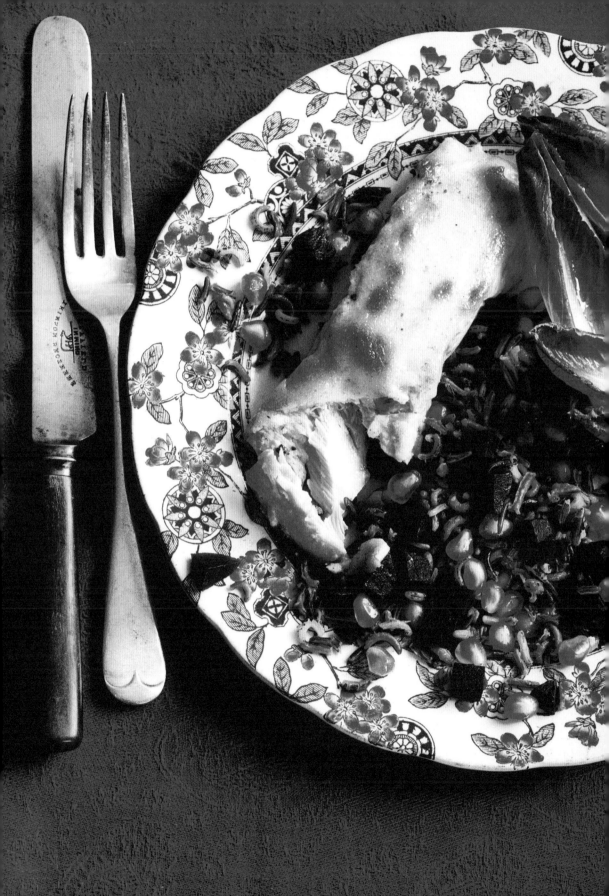

Salmon steaks with a wasabi coating

I adore the kick that wasabi gives to anything in its path. Buy it in powder form and add SLOWLY to dressings or mayonnaise, or if anyone you know goes to Japan, get them to bring you back some of the toxic green stuff in a tube.

Cook the wild rice (two parts water to one part rice) by boiling for 45 minutes. Leave to the side to cool.

Meanwhile, cover the beetroot/beet with water; bring to the boil, then reduce the heat and simmer for about 30 minutes until the beetroot/beet is tender. Drain, and when cool enough to handle, peel off the skin and cut the beetroot/beet into rough chunks.

Chop the pomegranate in half and extract the seeds. Add the pomegranate, beetroot/beet, olive oil and mint to the rice. Leave to the side.

Make the wasabi coating by mixing the mayonnaise, cumin and wasabi together. Taste and adjust if you want. Preheat the oven to 180°C/160°C fan/Gas 4.

Wash and dry the salmon, and season. Heat a griddle pan or ovenproof frying pan big enough to fit both salmon steaks and, when it is searing hot, drop the salmon in, skin-side down. Turn after 5 minutes or when the skin is brown and crispy. Take off the heat, carefully turn again, and spoon the wasabi mayonnaise onto the top of the salmon. Put the pan into the oven and cook for around 10 minutes until the glaze begins to brown. Serve on the wild rice.

SERVES 2

2 salmon steaks, about 175g/6oz each
Salt and pepper

For the rice

100g/¾ cup of wild rice
1 large beetroot/beet
1 pomegranate
1 tablespoon of olive oil
A small handful of fresh chopped mint

For the wasabi coating

2 tablespoons of mayonnaise
½ teaspoon of ground cumin
1 teaspoon of wasabi paste or powder mixed to a paste with water

Baked vegetables smothered in scamorza

SERVES 2

1 large aubergine/
   eggplant
Salt and pepper
2 tablespoons of olive oil
1 ball of smoked scamorza
   or smoked mozzarella
   (or use regular
   mozzarella)

For the pesto

1 large clove of
   garlic, peeled
A large handful of fresh
   basil
A few tablespoons of pine
   nuts
3 tablespoons of olive oil
30g/¼ cup of grated
   Parmesan
Salt and pepper

Scamorza is an Italian cow's milk cheese, available in most Italian delis. If you can't find it, use mozzarella instead. The smoked scamorza lends a smoky depth to sauces and whatever it touches. It is also pretty bloody good on it's own, eaten from the packet. This is a variation on a recipe given to me by my girlfriend Emma.

Preheat the oven to 180°C/160°C fan/Gas 4.

Start with salting the aubergine/eggplant. Slice it lengthways, put on a tea towel and sprinkle it with sea salt. Turn after 20 minutes or so, and do the other side. Rinse and dry thoroughly.

Make the pesto in a big pestle and mortar by grinding up the garlic. Add the basil, keep mashing away, and then add the pine nuts. Slowly add the olive oil, and then the Parmesan. Season to taste.

Put all the aubergine/eggplant in an ovenproof dish and give it a good dash of olive oil. Cook for around 10 minutes. Take out and spread the pesto on a layer of aubergine/eggplant, followed by a layer of scamorza or mozzarella (if using). Repeat the process until everything is used up. Bake for around 30 minutes and serve with a crisp green salad.

Root vegetable cakes with a cheesy béchamel sauce

Basically, a bubble-and-squeak cake with melted cheese on top. You could also serve this as an accompaniment to roast beef or any meat. Children seem to like these, they are crispy outside and sweet and moreish on the in. Serve with a gravy, either meat eaters or a mushroom or onion one for non-meat eaters.

To make the sauce, put the milk in a saucepan with the carrot, onion, parsley and peppercorns. Bring to the boil, turn down and simmer for 5 minutes. Pour the milk into a Pyrex jug. Wash the saucepan out and dry, then melt the butter. Slowly add the arrowroot, stirring continuously. Very slowly add the milk, again stirring all the while. When this is incorporated and smooth, add the cheese and stir until it melts. Season to taste and if too thick, add a few more drops of milk.

Bring all of the vegetables EXCEPT the spinach and leek to the boil in a pan of salted water, cooking until soft. This should take about 15 minutes. Take the pan off the heat and mash the vegetables roughly with a knob of butter and some salt and pepper.

In a separate pan, heat a knob of butter and soften the leek and spinach for a few minutes. Mix the spinach and leek into the coarsely mashed vegetables and form into small cakes. Pop in the fridge for an hour or so.

In a big frying pan, heat the olive oil. Put the cakes in and cook for a few minutes on each side, until they are lacy and golden. Serve with a big spoon of sauce.

SERVES 4

2 sweet potatoes, chopped into rough pieces
2 parsnips, chopped into rough pieces
2 carrots, chopped into rough pieces
A handful of chopped curly kale
½ a celeriac, chopped into small pieces
A handful of spinach, chopped
½ a leek, cut into small rounds
2 knobs of butter
Salt and pepper
2 tablespoons of olive oil

For the sauce
500ml/2 cups of milk
A few slices of carrot and onion
A few sprigs of fresh parsley
A few peppercorns
1 tablespoon of butter
1 tablespoon of arrowroot
50g/½ cup of grated cheese
Salt and pepper

Tofu lasagne

300g/1 block of firm tofu, drained, sliced across to make 1cm/½ inch thick rectangles (and patted dry with kitchen towel)
4 tablespoons of finely grated Parmesan
Salt and pepper
4 tablespoons of olive oil
4 portobello mushrooms, thickly sliced
200g/7oz of cherry tomatoes
2 cloves of garlic, peeled and finely sliced
3 tablespoons of balsamic vinegar
A handful of fresh basil leaves
2–3 fresh lasagne sheets per person

Something I used to make a lot when I lived in New York on a brisk night, that once again, even fussy children seem to like. If your carnivores are horrified by tofu, just substitute 400g/14oz of coarsely minced beef, and brown in a very hot pan with the olive oil. Instead of leaving to one side, carry on cooking with the sauce, and assemble as you would the original.

Coat the tofu in cheese, season generously and fry slices in 2 tablespoons of the oil until brown. Set aside. Fry the mushrooms in the remaining oil until browned, add the tomatoes and garlic and fry until the tomatoes are bursting. Add the balsamic and bubble down to caramelize. Throw in a splash of water along with the basil leaves to make a dressing. Stir and remove from the heat. Season with salt and pepper.

Cook the pasta according to the pack instructions. Drain in a colander and toss in a drizzle of olive oil to prevent the sheets sticking to each other. When just cool enough to handle, layer the pasta, tofu and mushroom mixture up on each plate, finishing with a couple of spoonfuls of the dressing in the pan and fresh basil leaves.

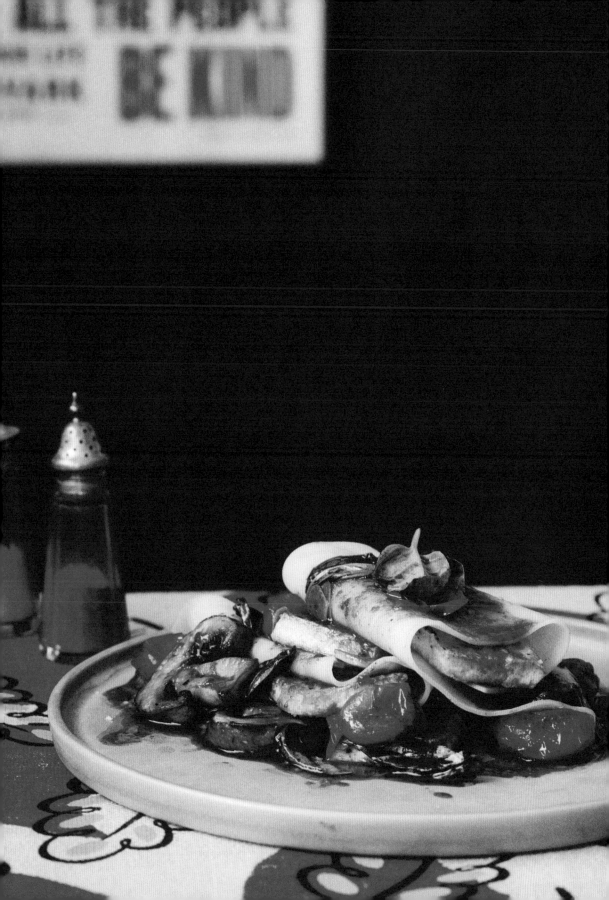

Chickpea/garbanzo bean mushroom burgers with tahini sauce

SERVES 4

2 tablespoons of olive oil

1 onion, peeled and finely chopped

2 cloves of garlic, peeled and finely chopped

500g/1lb 2oz of cooked and drained chickpeas/garbanzo beans

A handful of wild mushrooms, roughly torn

2 teaspoons of ground cumin

2 teaspoons of ground coriander

A small handful of fresh chopped parsley

3 tablespoons of spelt or plain/all-purpose flour

Salt and pepper

Hearty, and not at all worthy feeling, these are an easy thing to pull together if you have little time. They would also be good for a barbecue, woodsy and delicious.

Heat a frying pan and pour in a little olive oil. Add the onion and garlic and sweat for a few minutes. Keep to one side. Put all of the other ingredients in a blender and add the softened onion garlic mixture. Pulse until you have the consistency of breadcrumbs. Take the mixture out and fashion into burgers.

Heat some olive oil in a frying pan and cook the burgers for a few minutes on each side, until crispy and golden brown.

Mix the tahini sauce ingredients in a bowl and pour on top of the burgers. Eat with some minted rice or on a bun!

For the tahini sauce
3 tablespoons of olive oil
1 tablespoon of tahini
Juice of ½ a lemon

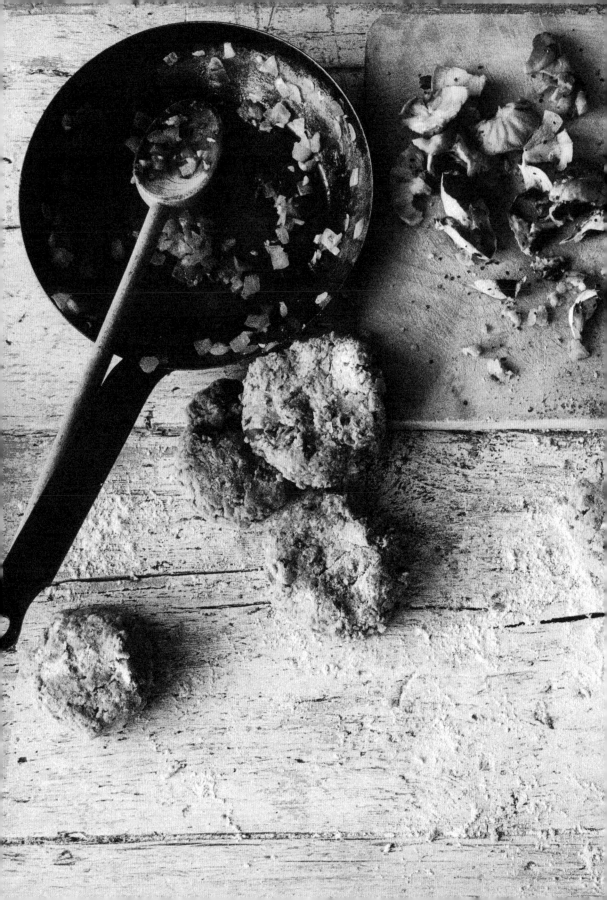

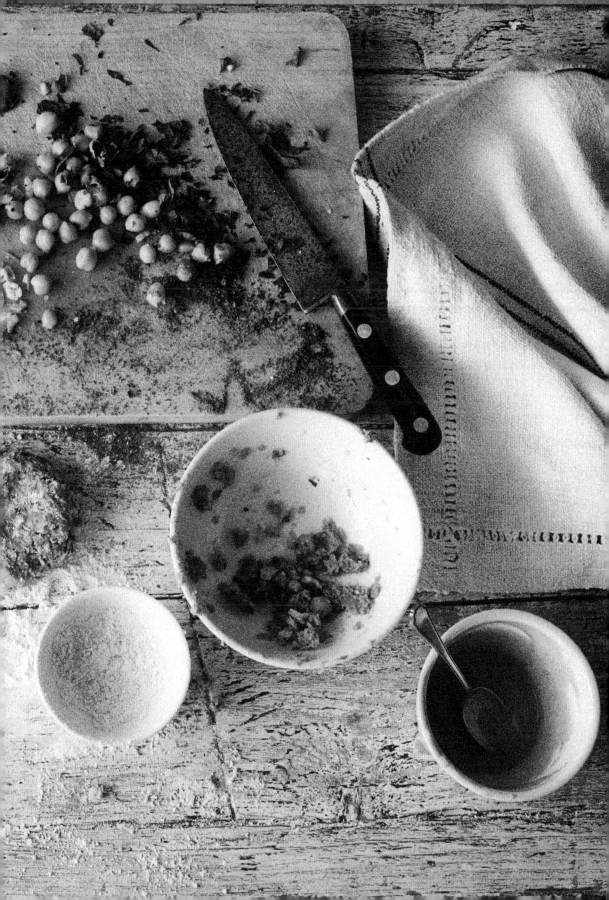

Lentil pie

You can leave this bare, top with a celeriac swede mash or colcannon, smother in cheese, or serve alongside rice. Whatever you do, eat it piping hot, with lots of peas on the side, and possibly some tomato ketchup.

Place the lentils in a pan and add just enough water to cover. Simmer over a low heat for 20 minutes, then drain.

In a large frying pan, heat the olive oil. Throw in the onion and the garlic and cook on a low heat until soft. Add the carrots and cook for another few minutes. Add the tomatoes and celery, followed by the red wine, then the stock, the Worcestershire sauce, Tabasco and the bay leaves. Stir it all the while. Add the balsamic vinegar and also the parsley. Leave for another few minutes, and then add the lentils. Cook for a few minutes and serve in bowls, with a dollop of crème fraîche, some more parsley and perhaps some spinach.

SERVES 4

100g/½ cup of Puy lentils

2 tablespoons of olive oil

1 large red onion, peeled and finely chopped

2 cloves of garlic, peeled and crushed

2 large carrots, chopped quite small

200g/1 cup of canned plum tomatoes

2 celery sticks, chopped

1 small glass of red wine

600ml/2½ cups of vegetable stock

1 tablespoon of Worcestershire sauce, or to taste

A few drops of Tabasco sauce

A few bay leaves

A teaspoon of syrupy balsamic vinegar

A small handful of fresh parsley

1 tablespoon of crème fraîche/sour cream

The first Mor Mor and her chicken

My great-grandmother, a Norwegian, Sofie Magdalene Hesselberg, was known as the first Mor Mor in my family. 'Mor Mor' is an affectionate moniker used by grandchildren in many Scandinavian countries, referring to their 'mother's mother'.

Sofie was a tough cookie. Having emigrated in her early twenties from Norway to Wales, she lost her husband and eldest daughter within a few months of each other, and was left in a foreign country with three small children of her own and two stepchildren to take care of. A lesser woman would have been felled. Mor Mor got on with it, fulfilling her late husband's wishes of putting all his children through the British school system, and managing to keep a staunch sense of humour and practicality during what must have been a shattering time. She told her children Norse legends about trolls, fjord dwelling spirits and fairies. She also smoked cigars and had a crystal ball. I wish I had known her.

One of her daughters remembers her making the following during the war, when they lived near a farmer who would sometimes donate them a chicken on the sly. It has been passed down, and here it is.

Place the chicken in a large casserole and pour the chicken stock over it until it is nearly covered. Add a quarter of the carrots, the onions, bouquet garni and bay leaf and bring to the boil. When it has boiled, turn it right down and simmer on a very low heat for 2 hours. One hour and forty minutes in, add the remaining carrots and all the potatoes, and top up with more stock if needs be. About 3 minutes before the 2 hour mark, add the peas.

Take the chicken and vegetables out of the casserole and leave to the side. Take the remaining juices in the casserole and strain as a stock for the sauce.

Melt the butter in a pan, gently add the flour and cook on a low heat for a few minutes. Add the stock, bit by bit, stirring continuously. Season to taste, and then start gently adding the milk. Cook for several minutes.

Hopefully your chicken will be cool enough to touch. Remove all the flesh from the carcass and get rid of the skin. Put the chicken and vegetables back in the casserole, cover in the sauce and heat gently. Serve with some parsley.

SERVES 4–6

1 medium-sized happy
  free-range chicken
1.2 litres/5 cups of chicken
  stock
700g/1½lb carrots
2 medium onions, peeled
  and finely sliced
A bouquet garni
1 bay leaf
200g/7oz of potatoes, cut
  into rough chunks
225g/1½ cups of frozen
  peas
50g/½ stick of butter
50g/scant ½ cup of
  plain/all-purpose flour
Salt and pepper
300ml/1¼ cups of milk
A handful of fresh
  chopped parsley

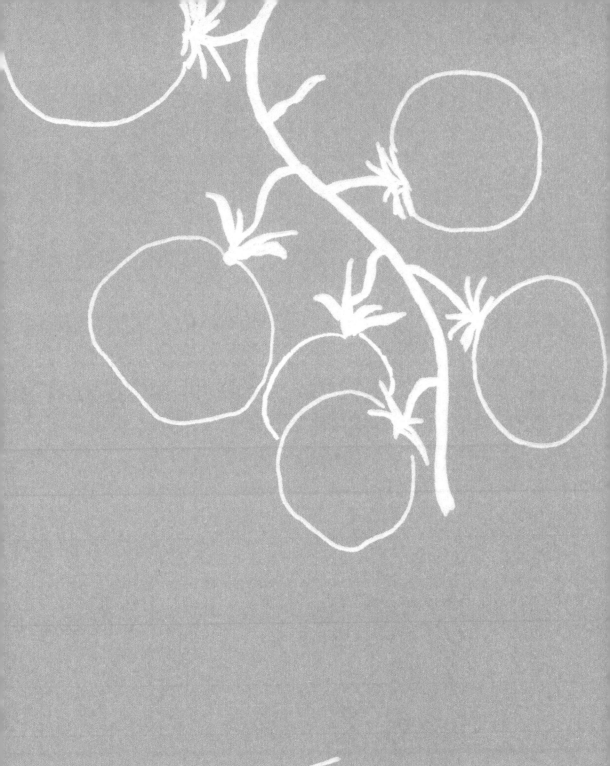

Vine Tomatoes

Winter

BREAKFASTS
Dosa
Aloo gobi
Soda bread with goat's curd and blistered tomatoes
Mexican eggs
Porridge with poached plums
Warming winter take on miso soup
Poached pears with healthy vanilla custard

LUNCHES
Cauliflower chowder and a brilliant bread recipe
Taleggio gratin
Stuffed blini and scrambled eggs
Salad of brown rice and pearl barley with cranberries
Watercress and Gruyère soufflé
Endive salad with poached duck eggs and truffle vinaigrette
Quiche with crispy back bacon and caramelized onions

SUPPERS
Winter curry with saffron cinnamon rice
Penne with almond goat's curd parsley pesto
Fish fingers with tartare sauce and mushy peas
Overnight lamb
Vegetable and chicken itame (or an honest stir-fry to the uniniated!)
Halibut with sorrel sauce and Jerusalem artichoke purée
The second Mor Mor's chicken

Winter breakfasts and dancing pigeons

Amongst the many odd things I have done, none was odder than my turn, many years ago, as a leading lady in a Bollywood film. I was unspeakably bad in it and it cured me of any latent desire to be an actress. I should also think it cured anyone watching of the desire to ever see me act again. However, I can lip synch in Hindi whilst dancing with bells on my ankles, which may one day come in very useful.

I am not a natural synchronized dancer. I am incredibly graceless and can't follow instructions. I remember being struck dumb with terror and embarrassment as a bevy of Bollywood lovelies, backing dancers, stood behind me, rolling their eyes as I tried to pick up some simple step. The terror was exacerbated one day when I came to work to dance barefoot and was confronted by a very large rustling crate that seemed to coo and scratch and breathe.

'What is in that crate?' I asked.

'Oh, it's the dancing pigeons,' the director replied, breezily. 'Five hundred of them. They will dance around your feet, whilst you dance. It will be one big happy dance party. Yeah!'

Reader, I hate pigeons. I loathe and abhor them. I hate them in the sky, but I hate them more if they are 'dancing' with their scabby, prehistoric feet, next to my own clumsy, enormous, BARE feet in an echoing sound stage in Mumbai.

'Are you bloody joking?' I said with mounting panic. 'You want me to dance barefoot in the midst of five hundred pigeons?! And look like a joyful village belle?'

'Yes,' the director said, with a steely look, one I could not face arguing with.

I 'danced' with a veil in the middle of a sea of five hundred pigeons. There is a look of maniacal fear on my face, as I navigated around pigeon droppings and small claws, remembering to lip synch in Hindi and not count time out – loud. I think it took about ten hours, although it felt like a lifetime. Those bastard pigeons didn't make the final cut.

Having spent a few solitary months in Mumbai, I also became particularly partial to an Indian breakfast. I was very lonely, and it was the highlight of my day. I made friends with the room service waiter, Akesh, who every morning seemed disappointed that I had not morphed into the screen siren Aishwarya Rai overnight. His eyes fell when he saw it was still dreary me in my pyjamas, a Bollywood pretender. So to him I apologize, but to you I say, dosa recipes are far more useful than tinkling ankles and making friends with pigeons.

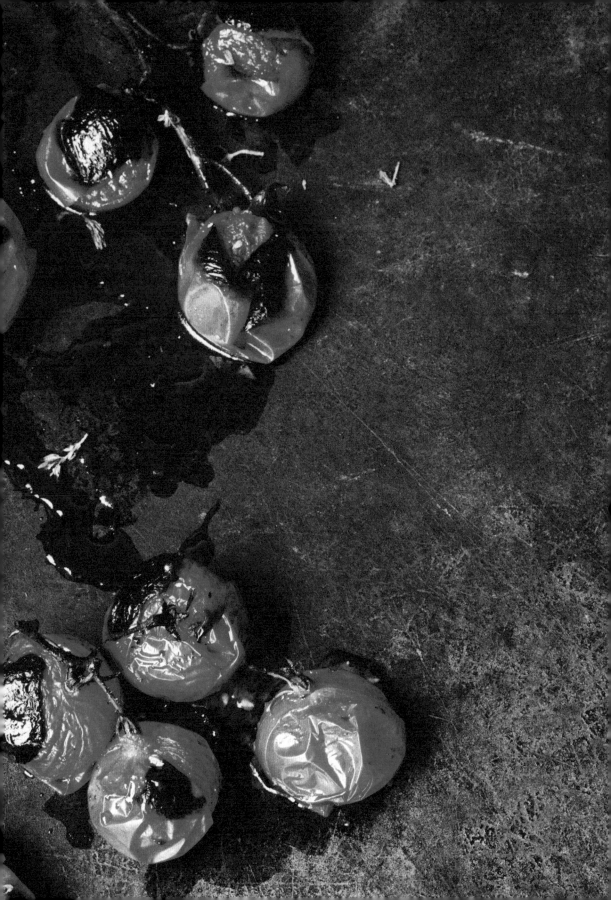

Winter
Breakfasts

Dosa

SERVES 4–6
90g/½ cup of rice flour
60g/½ cup of semolina
60ml/¼ cup of wholemilk
   plain yoghurt
A handful of fresh
   chopped
   coriander/cilantro
2 tablespoons of
   sunflower oil or ghee

An easy yoghurt dosa batter for an Indian breakfast with aloo gobi and chutney.

In a large mixing bowl, mix the flour and semolina with the yoghurt, the coriander/cilantro and 250ml (1 cup) of water. Cover the bowl and leave on the side for a few hours. You may need to add a few spoons of water just before cooking, as the flour will thicken and suck up all the liquid in sight! You want a thin batter consistency, but not so thin that it sticks to the pan.

Heat a non-stick griddle pan and brush with the oil or ghee. Make one test dosa by pouring a ladleful of batter into the pan, trying to keep it as evenly dispersed and thin as possible. When it is bubbling and pinpricked, turn it and cook the other side for a minute or two. Hopefully you've found your formula and the rest will be a breeze. Serve immediately with aloo gobi and some chutney.

Aloo gobi

Heat the oil or ghee in a heavy-bottomed pan. Add the chopped onion and cook on a medium heat until softened. Add the spices, chilli and curry leaves and mix together, cooking for a few minutes. Next, add the tomatoes and potatoes with the water, bring to the boil, reducing the heat slightly and letting it cook on low for around 10 to 15 minutes. Then add the cauliflower, the sugar, lemon and cinnamon, stir it all in, adding a little more water if it is looking dry, and cook for another 10 to 15 minutes. Season to taste.

This is even more delicious the next day, after a night in the fridge, liberally covered in chopped coriander/cilantro.

SERVES 3–4

2 tablespoons of sunflower oil or ghee

1 small onion, finely chopped

½ teaspoon of ground coriander

½ teaspoon of ground turmeric

½ teaspoon of ground ginger

1 teaspoon of mustard seeds

1 small green chilli, deseeded (or not, according to your heat tolerance) and finely chopped

A few curry leaves

250g/1 cup of chopped tomatoes (fresh or canned)

4 medium potatoes, peeled and quartered

About 6 tablespoons of water

½ a small head of cauliflower, broken up into florets

½ teaspoon of sugar

1 teaspoon of lemon juice

A pinch of ground cinnamon

Salt and pepper

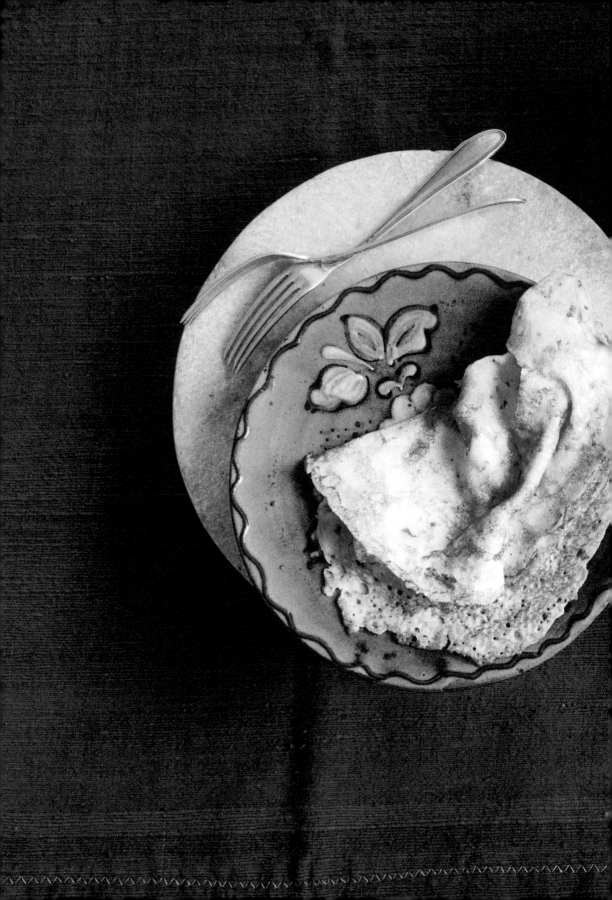

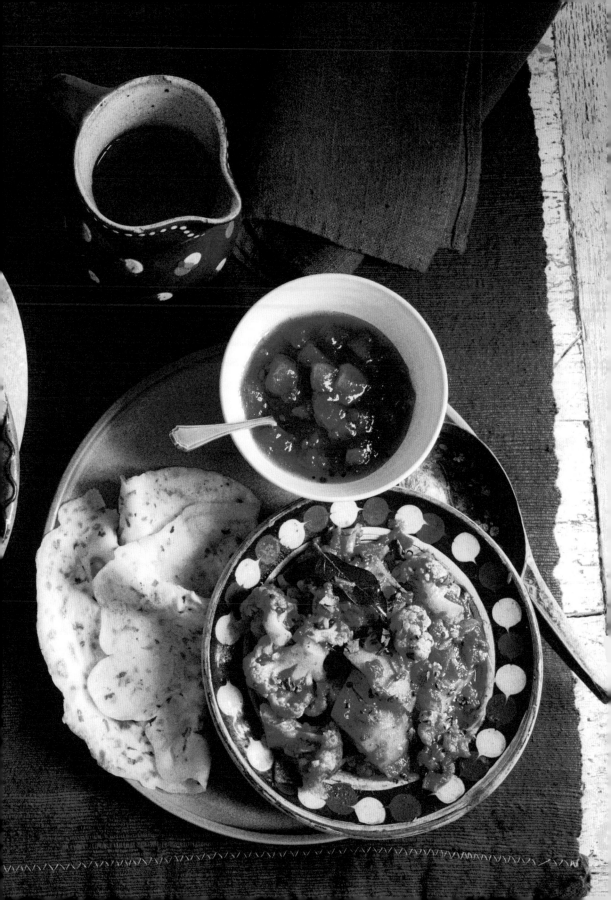

Soda bread with goat's curd and blistered tomatoes

SERVES 2

For the soda bread
400g/3 cups of
   stoneground
   wholemeal/whole
   wheat flour or plain/all-
   purpose white flour (I've
   also used spelt and that
   works too)
1 teaspoon of bicarbonate
   of soda/baking soda
1 teaspoon of salt
350ml/1⅓ cups of
   buttermilk

Soda bread is so easy, and discovering the ease of it makes the world of bread making suddenly seem far less frightening and more accessible. This is a gorgeous wintry breakfast, made better still with a bit of olive oil and a pinch of sea salt.

Preheat the oven to 200°C/180°C fan/Gas 6.

In a large mixing bowl, mix the dry ingredients together and make a well in the centre of the bowl with your hand. Pour all of the buttermilk into the well and, using your hand, mix the flour into the buttermilk in a circular motion, from the well to the sides, so you draw all the flour into the middle. You want the dough soft, but not too sticky or elastic. This shouldn't take long and you don't want to meddle around with the dough too much. Put the dough onto a floured surface or board.

Give the dough a gentle roll with your hands to shape it into a ball and turn it over. Place it on a floured baking tray, cut a deep cross in the middle, and put it in the oven. Bake for 40 minutes. If you're not sure if it's ready, tap the base, which should sound hollow.

To make the blistered tomatoes, preheat the grill to very hot. Wash and dry the tomatoes, taking care to keep their vine intact. Pop them in a roasting tin, season, pour on a glug of both the olive oil and balsamic vinegar and then sprinkle with the thyme. Grill for about 5 to 10 minutes or until their skins are just beginning to break and char.

Smear your bread with goat's curd or cheese, curl your tomatoes up by it, and spoil it all by mashing them into the cheesy bread and eating. Yum.

For the blistered tomatoes
Tomatoes on the vine, about 12–16 for 2 people
Salt and pepper
A glug of olive oil
A glug of good thick balsamic vinegar (I use white, but any will do)
A tablespoon or so of fresh chopped thyme
50g/½ cup of goat's curd or a soft goat's cheese

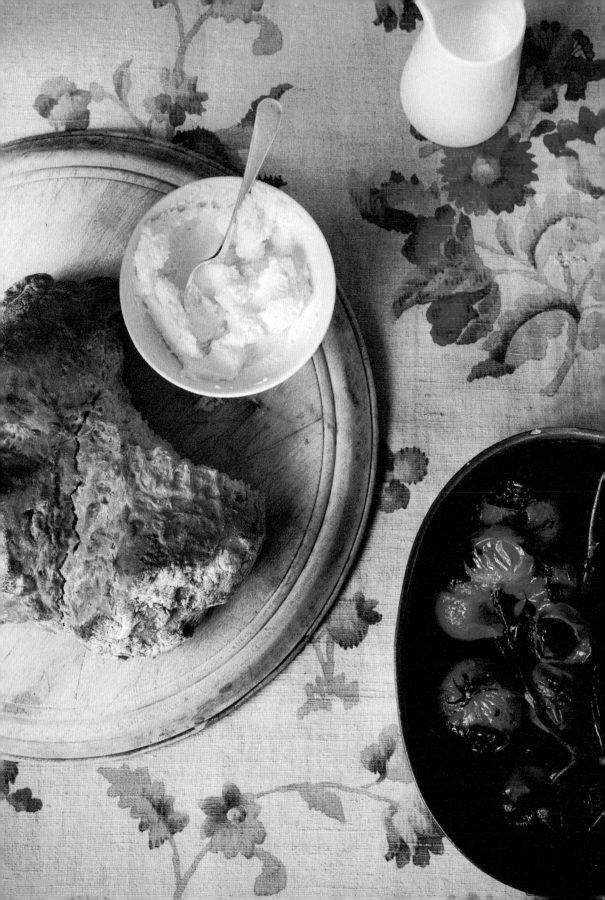

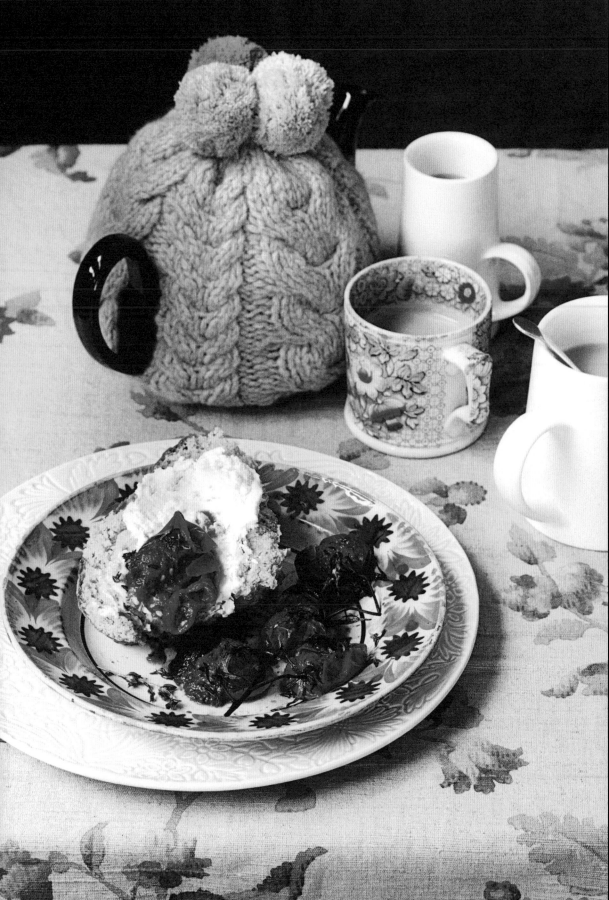

Mexican eggs

SERVES 2

1 tablespoon of either
   butter or olive oil
½ an onion, peeled and
   finely chopped
2 tomatoes, finely chopped
1 small green chilli,
   deseeded and finely
   chopped
4 eggs
50g/½ cup of Queso Fresco
   (crumbly Mexican
   cheese) or Manchego,
   crumbled or grated
Salt and pepper
A small handful of fresh
   finely chopped
   coriander/cilantro

Who cares if we're stuck in England in December?
We have these eggs to remind us of the faraway, and
they're a lot cheaper than a return flight to Cabo.
Serve with some spicy hot chocolate. (Add a
cinnamon stick and a pinch of dried red chilli to your
hot chocolate pan and leave to infuse on low for a
few minutes.)

On a lowish heat, melt the butter or oil in a heavy-bottomed frying
pan. Add the onion and cook for a few minutes, and then add the
tomatoes and chilli and give a good stir. Whilst these are cooking,
whisk the eggs into the mixture, stirring gently all the while as you
would with scrambled eggs.

Add the cheese at the last moment, season to taste and serve
liberally with coriander/cilantro unless you are my brother-in-law, Ben
Cullum, who has a mortal loathing of the stuff. I like this smothered
with Tabasco sauce with a bowl of guacamole on the side.

Porridge with poached plums

I could quite happily eat porridge every day. Cold, too, with honey. I could be hired as the fourth bear.

Soak the porridge oats overnight in a cup (250ml) full of water. Leave to the side, covered with a tea towel. When you wake up, pour the oats into a saucepan and bring to the boil with another 500ml/ 2 cups of water. When you have it at a rolling boil, turn down the heat, add a pinch of salt and simmer on low for around 45 minutes.

Whilst your porridge is cooking, make the poached plums. Put the plums in a saucepan, cover with the water, and add the agave or sugar and the spices. Bring to the boil and then simmer until the fruit is soft, about 5 or so minutes.

Serve the porridge with a generous juicy tablespoon of the plums and their juice. If you want to be very decadent, add a lick of cream.

SERVES 4

100g/1 cup of porridge
   oats (slow cooking, like
   McCann's)
A pinch of salt

For the plums
450g/1lb of plums, stoned
   and quartered
4 tablespoons of agave
   syrup or brown sugar
1 cinnamon stick
A few cloves

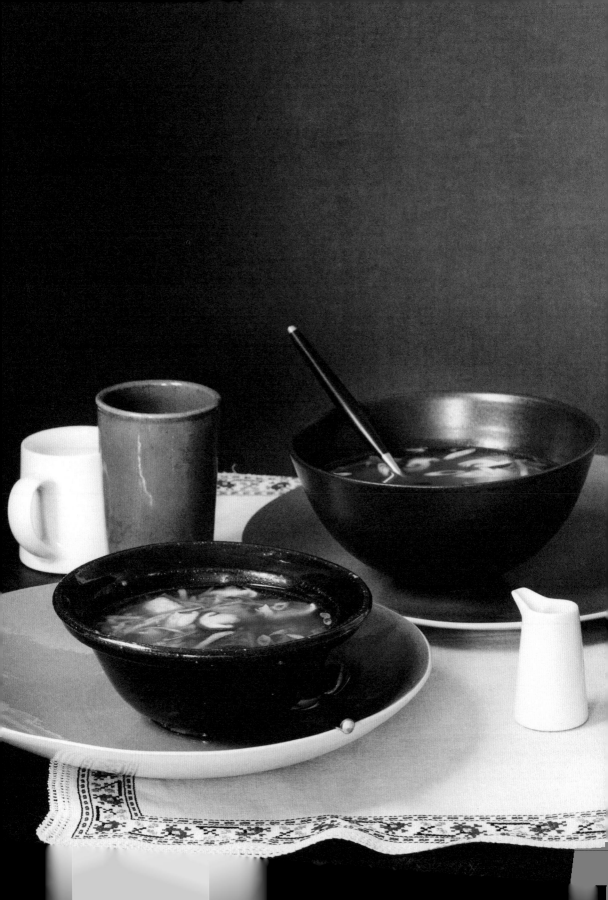

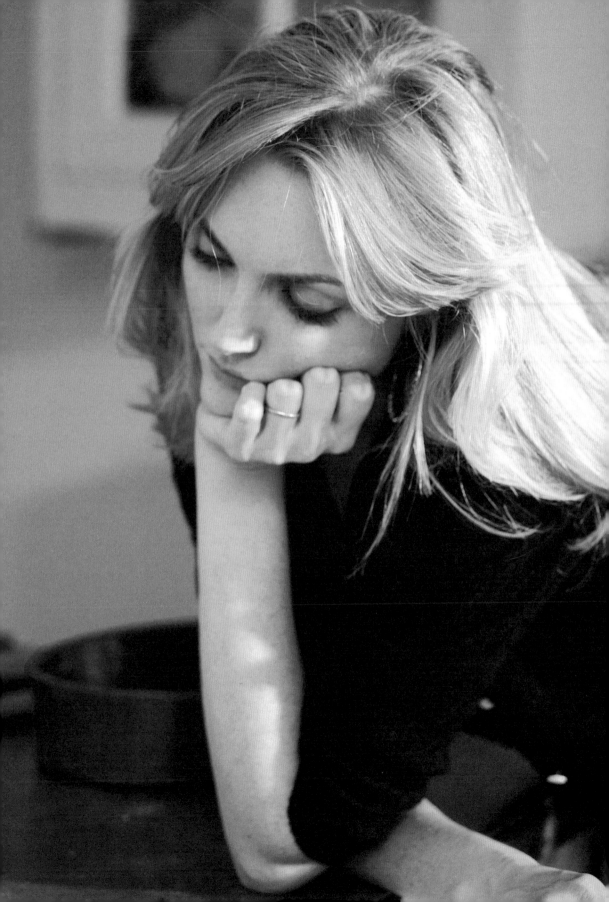

Warming winter take on miso soup

SERVES 1

400ml/1½ cups of
  vegetable stock
1 carrot, coarsely grated
4 shiitake mushrooms,
  quartered
1 parsnip, coarsely grated
½ an onion, peeled and
  thinly sliced in half-
  moon shapes
150g/½ a block of firm tofu,
  drained and patted dry
  with kitchen towel
1 tablespoon of sesame oil
1–2 tablespoons of barley
  miso paste (most health
  shops should stock this)
1 spring onion/scallion,
  finely chopped

Another breakfast friend discovered during my weird nomadic former career, earthy miso soup. Of course it should be served at breakfast time, try it and see. It makes total sense. I would have it with a little bowl of rice and some pickles.

In a medium-sized saucepan, pour in the stock and add the grated carrot, mushrooms, parsnip and onion and bring to the boil. Reduce the heat and cook on low for about 15 to 20 minutes.

Cut the tofu into small cubes and, in a separate frying pan, heat the oil and cook the tofu until it is golden brown. Drain the oil and add the tofu to the soup. Mix the miso paste with a couple of spoonfuls of broth and pour it into the pan. Give it a good stir. Add the chopped spring onion/scallion to serve.

Poached pears with healthy vanilla custard

Obviously custard is good made with ladles of cream and sugar, this we know. But at breakfast time, this may be pushing it and your blood sugar levels. This way is still perfectly respectable.

Make sure you have a shallow pan that all your pears will fit in. Put the apple juice, agave or honey, cinnamon stick and star anise into the pan and bring to the boil, stirring it to incorporate the agave. When bubbling, turn the heat down, add the pears and cook on a low to medium heat for about 10 minutes. When the pears are soft, turn the heat off and leave to the side.

For the custard, pour the milk into a saucepan and scrape the insides of the vanilla pod/bean into it. Heat the milk until it begins to bubble, and then take off the heat. In a mixing bowl, whisk together the egg yolks, the arrowroot and the syrup, and when combined, slowly whisk the warm milk in. Strain the custard into a clean pan and heat on low, whisking until the custard is thick and warm. Serve on top of the pears.

SERVES 4

For the pears
500ml/2 cups of apple juice
4 tablespoons of agave syrup or honey
1 cinnamon stick
1 star anise
4 pears, peeled, cored and halved

For the custard
300ml/1¼ cups of semi-skimmed milk
1 vanilla pod/bean
2 egg yolks
2 teaspoons of arrowroot
4 tablespoons of maple or agave syrup

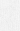

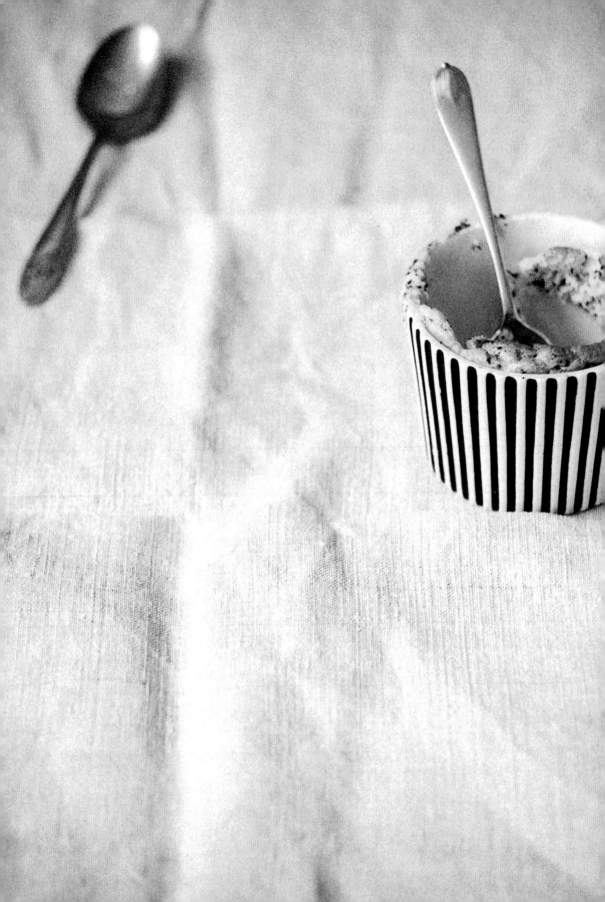

Winter
Lunches

Cauliflower chowder and a brilliant bread recipe

SERVES 3–4

For the bread

A small handful each of
poppy seeds, sunflower
seeds and pumpkin
seeds

450g/3 cups of
wholemeal/whole
wheat flour

115g/1 cup of spelt flour

2 tablespoons of brown
sugar

1 teaspoon or a large pinch
of salt

1 egg

500ml/2 cups of plain
yoghurt

1 tablespoon of olive oil

On the twisting road halfway between San Francisco and Big Sur in lashing rain, my friend and I came across a farm stand, like a mirage. There was cauliflower chowder on a hot plate, home-made bread and butter, chocolate chip cookies and beautiful peaches. There was no one serving, you put your money in a glass jar. We sat in contented silence, our soup in paper cups, bread in our hands, thanking the day we were born. This is an ode to that day.

Grease a loaf tin and sprinkle the inside with an even coating of poppy seeds. Mix the flours, sugar and salt together in a big mixing bowl and separately mix the egg, yoghurt and olive oil in a large Pyrex (or something similar) jug. Gently add the wet to the dry, mixing well. Your dough should feel sticky and damp. Sprinkle over the other seeds. Place it in the prepared loaf tin and leave it in a warm place for 2 hours.

Preheat the oven to 180°C/160°C fan/Gas 4. Bake the loaf in the oven for 1 hour or so, and then take it out and check that it makes a hollow sound when you tip it out of the loaf tin and tap the base. Place on a wire rack to cool.

For the soup, Heat the olive oil or butter in a big heavy-bottomed pan on a low to medium heat. Add the onion, potatoes and celery and cook for a few minutes. Pour in the chicken stock and half of the milk.

Add the cauliflower and flake the haddock into the soup, topping up with milk if needed. Simmer for about 15 minutes, slowly adding the rest of the milk, and add the cream shortly before you serve. Season and give it a generous handful of parsley. Serve with the bread.

For the chowder

1 tablespoon of olive oil or butter
1 onion, peeled and finely chopped
2 potatoes, diced
2 celery sticks, finely diced
600ml/2½ cups of chicken stock (preferably fresh free-range chicken stock)
250ml/1 cup of milk
1 small head of cauliflower, broken up into small florets
1 large fillet of undyed smoked haddock
3 tablespoons of single/light cream
Salt and pepper
A handful of fresh chopped parsley

Taleggio gratin

You can play around with this using different types of vegetables, but nothing that gets too watery or it becomes a running mess. Do drain the spinach properly and squash all the excess water out.

Start with the sauce. Melt the butter in a saucepan and whisk in the flour. Pour in the milk, whisking constantly until it starts to boil. Season, reduce the heat and simmer on low for about 10 minutes. Remove from the heat and taste, adding a pinch of nutmeg, if you like it. Add more milk if it is too thick.

Sprinkle the celeriac with a little salt to season. Put half the butter in a large saucepan, add the celeriac and cook on a medium heat for 5 or so minutes, stirring it. Add a tablespoon of water, cover the pan and cook the celeriac until it's tender, about 15 minutes.

In a small saucepan, heat the olive oil and add the onion, cooking on low for 10 minutes, or until soft. Add the spinach, season, and cook for another 3 minutes or so to wilt. Drain.

Preheat the oven to 200°C/180°C fan/Gas 6 and grease an ovenproof dish with half a tablespoon of olive oil.

Put a layer of the celeriac into your ovenproof dish and cover with the spinach and onion and then a layer of béchamel. Sprinkle the Taleggio on top. Carry on this process in layers until all of your ingredients are used up, ending with a layer of cheese-sprinkled béchamel. Bake for 20 minutes or until golden and bubbling.

SERVES 4

For the béchamel sauce
4 tablespoons of butter
40g/⅓ cup of plain/all-purpose flour
580ml/2½ cups of milk
Salt and pepper
A pinch of freshly grated nutmeg (optional)

For the gratin
4 celeriac (about 2kg/4½lb), peeled, halved and thinly sliced
Salt and pepper
3 tablespoons of butter
2 tablespoons olive oil
1 small onion, peeled and thinly sliced
450g/1lb of spinach, washed and roughly chopped
60g/½ cup of grated Taleggio cheese

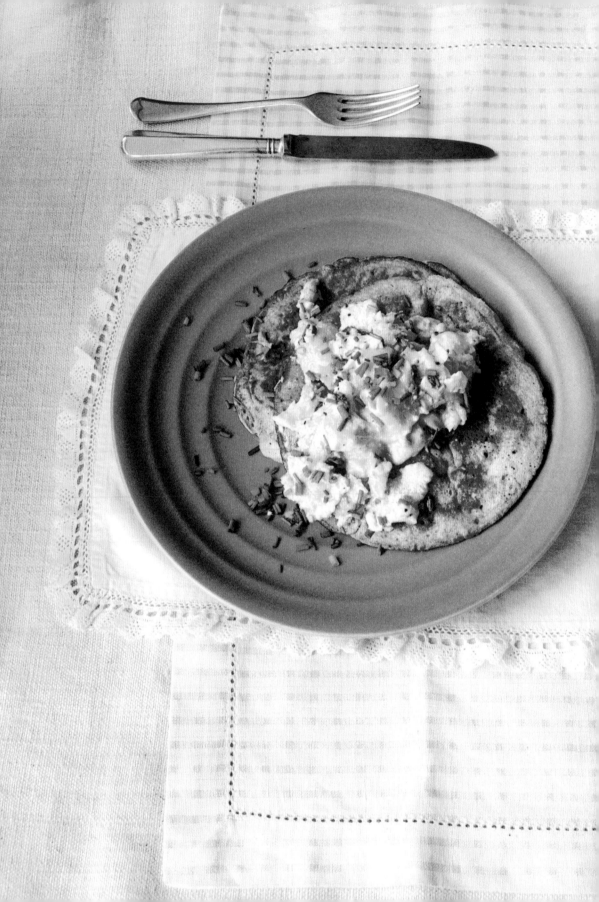

Stuffed blini and scrambled eggs

I made this on New Year's Eve for a few people in my kitchen. It's that perfect combination of treat and comfort and works as a weekend breakfast, lunch or dinner. You can use any cheese or herb combination that takes your fancy, Cheddar and chive is also good, with a bit of mustard powder, as is Parmesan with some very thinly sliced sun-dried tomato chucked in. Even though it is simple, it feels a ceremony.

In a large mixing bowl, sift in the flour, baking powder and a pinch of salt and whisk well with the milk to make a batter. Add the ricotta, chives and parsley and mix again. In a separate clean bowl, whisk the egg whites until they form soft peaks. Fold them gently into the batter mixture, being careful not to over mix.

In a small frying pan (preferably non-stick), heat a little butter or olive oil and spoon in a ladleful of the batter to cover the pan. Cook for 3 to 4 minutes until pinprick bubbles appear and you can turn easily. Cook the other side for a minute or so, continuing until all the batter is used up. If you are a great multitasker, you can make the scrambled eggs at the same time. If not, pop the blini in a warm oven while you're making the eggs.

To make the scrambled eggs, whisk the eggs and egg yolks and season. In a medium-sized pan, heat a knob of butter on a low heat. Add the eggs, stirring continuously and adding a little milk if they are dry. After a minute or so, take off the heat and continue to stir as the eggs will cook themselves. Put a blini (or two) on each plate and serve covered in scrambled eggs and any chopped herbs you have left over.

SERVES 4

For the blini
175g/1½ cups of buckwheat flour
2 teaspoons of baking powder
A pinch of salt
300ml/1¼ cups of milk
150g/½ cup of ricotta cheese, crumbled
A small handful of fresh finely chopped chives and parsley
4 egg whites (you can use the yolks for the scrambled eggs)
A knob of butter or spoon of olive oil

For the scrambled eggs
2 eggs
4 egg yolks
Salt and pepper
A knob of butter
A dash of milk (optional)

Salad of brown rice and pearl barley with cranberries

SERVES 6–8

2 tablespoons of olive oil

1 small onion, peeled and
  finely chopped

200g/1 cup of brown rice,
  rinsed

200g/1 cup of pearl barley,
  rinsed

A pinch of salt

½ a red cabbage, finely
  shredded

1 celery stick, finely diced

A handful of dried
  cranberries

A handful of fresh
  chopped parsley

A handful of pecans

For the dressing

1 tablespoon of red wine
  vinegar

3 tablespoons of olive oil

1 shallot peeled and finely
  chopped

A handful of fresh finely
  chopped thyme

Salt and pepper

A colourful salad filled with goodness and complex aminos. Dried cranberries are marvellous and are readily available in most supermarkets and health food shops. You could add some toasted walnuts or almonds to this. You can also swap a grain for another: red rice, couscous, the possibilities are many.

In a large saucepan, heat the olive oil. Add the onion and sweat for a few minutes, and then stir in the grains. Double the water to the grains, adding a pinch of salt, and bring to the boil. When boiling, reduce the heat, and simmer on low for around 30 to 40 minutes.

When the grains have cooled, transfer to a salad bowl and add the shredded cabbage, celery, cranberries and the parsley. Toast the pecans in a small frying pan for a few minutes and add to the salad.

Mix the dressing and pour over the salad. Serve.

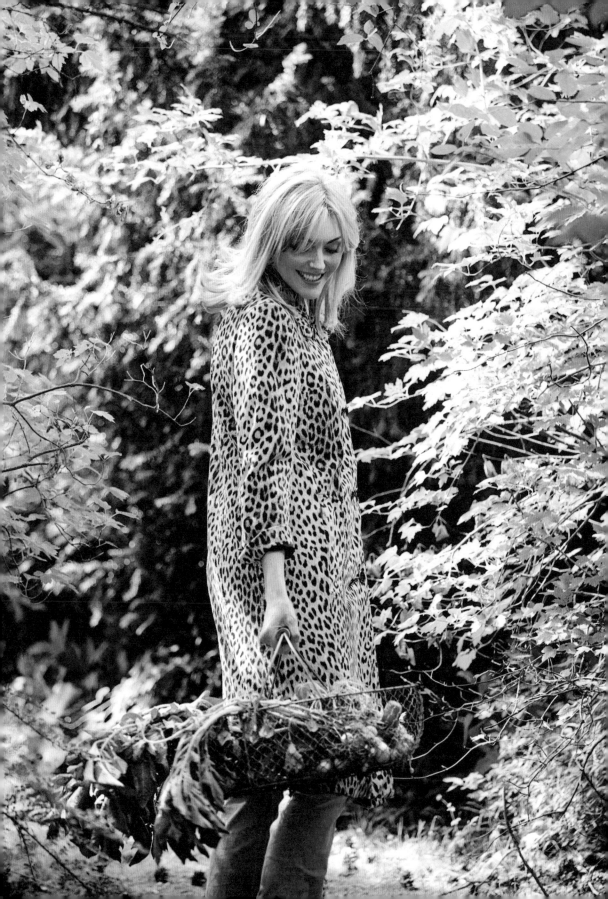

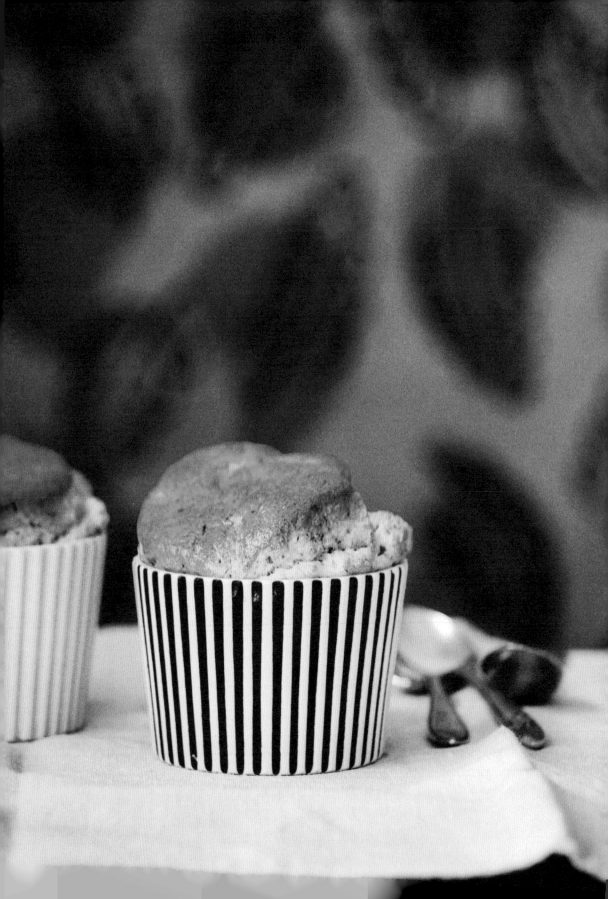

Watercress and Gruyère soufflé

The mere mention of the word 'soufflé' has historically been enough to strike fear into the hearts of those who are ordinarily hardy in the kitchen. In the face of that golden mountain of unpredictability, many are rendered quivering wrecks. The soufflé is the bad boy of the kitchen, the one whose negative traits are legend. This character, which others warn us about, is unstable and liable to burn us. It's reputation seems a bit unfair – a vulnerable artistic type, yes, but in the flesh, oh how rewarding, complex and delicious.

I'll give you a case in point for the defence. A thirteen-year-old me, bored, on a rainy Saturday, finding a soufflé recipe in an old cookbook of my mum's. We had eggs, flour, cheese and butter in the house, so I thought I'd give it a go. Nobody was there to shake a head, or tell me how difficult it was going to be. So I made one. It came out of the oven, high and beautiful, a perfect illustration of the heady alchemy that goes on in cooking. My mum came home from the shops, or tarot card reader, or wherever she was, and was shocked to the core.

'You made a soufflé!' She cried.

'Yeah.' I said. 'So?'

Cut to years later, a twenty-one-year-old me, poisoned by years of meddling warnings from cookery shows and books, cooking a soufflé for a boyfriend (and six friends) who I was showing off to.

2 tablespoons of unsalted
   butter, plus softened
   butter to coat the
   ramekins
230g/2 cups of grated
   Gruyère
I small bunch (50g/2oz) of
   watercress, tough stalks
   removed
30g/¼ cup of plain/
   all-purpose flour
300ml/1¼ cups of semi-
   skimmed milk
6 eggs, separated
Salt and pepper
A pinch of nutmeg

It came out of the oven a flat, miserable, eggy mess, which reduced my boasting and I to shreds.

The moral of the story is, don't be swayed by other people's experience. Experiment with the cool of a child.

Preheat the oven to 200°C/180°C fan/Gas 6. Grease six 250ml/1 cup ramekins with the softened butter and then coat with 30g/¼ cup of the cheese. Place the ramekins on a baking tray and chill in the fridge.

Blanch the watercress quickly in a pan of boiling water, remove immediately and plunge into ice water, and then squeeze all of the water out. Stick it in the blender and purée or chop very finely, then leave it on the side.

Melt the rest of the butter in a pan over a low heat and add the flour to make a roux, stirring continuously for about a minute. Gently add the milk, bit by bit, still stirring constantly. Let the sauce bubble for a minute or two and add the remaining cheese. Continue stirring until all the cheese has melted. Remove from the heat and leave to cool for a few minutes, then stir in the egg yolks and season, adding at this point the puréed watercress and a pinch of nutmeg.

In a separate very clean bowl, whisk the egg whites and a pinch of salt until they form stiff peaks. Fold half of this mix gently into the cheese watercress roux until combined, taking care not to overly mix as you want to keep it airy. Repeat this with the other half of the egg whites.

Divide the mixture evenly into the ramekins and level the tops with a spatula. Run the tip of your thumb around the inside of each dish to make a gap between the soufflé and the dish, which will help it to rise. Place the dishes on the baking tray and bake for at least 15 minutes, possibly more. DON'T open the oven to check – resist the urge, however great. They will collapse. When they are golden and majestic, serve immediately and, if they should collapse, you must not. Laugh instead.

Endive salad with poached duck eggs and truffle vinaigrette

Duck eggs are rich, gamey and largely unsung. They poach beautifully and, paired with the crisp endive and earthy truffle, they are total bliss. My mum used to fry them for breakfast.

Wash and trim the ends off the endive. Dry and lay on four plates. In a small frying pan, toast the walnuts on a medium heat for a few minutes.

Make the dressing by whisking together the truffle oil, shallot, vinegar, lemon juice and salt and pepper. Adjust to taste.

Bring some water to a simmer in a pan with a splash of vinegar and salt. Carefully add the duck eggs and poach for 3 minutes. Drain and put on top of the endive, with a handful of walnuts and the dressing spooned on.

SERVES 4

1 endive per person
1 handful of walnuts, chopped
A splash of white wine vinegar
Salt
4 duck eggs

For the dressing

2 tablespoons of truffle oil
½ shallot, peeled and finely chopped
1¼ teaspoons of champagne vinegar or white wine vinegar
A quick squeeze of lemon juice
Salt and pepper

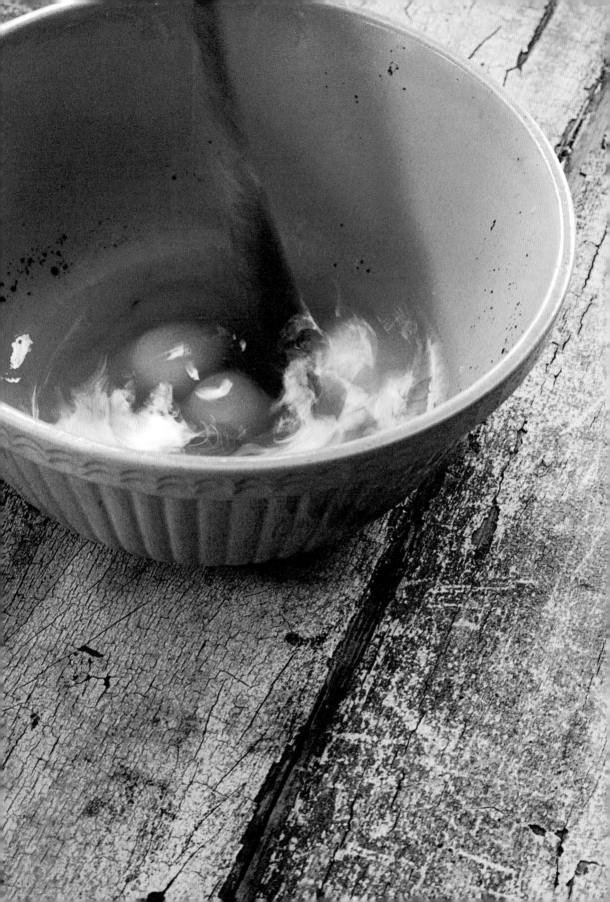

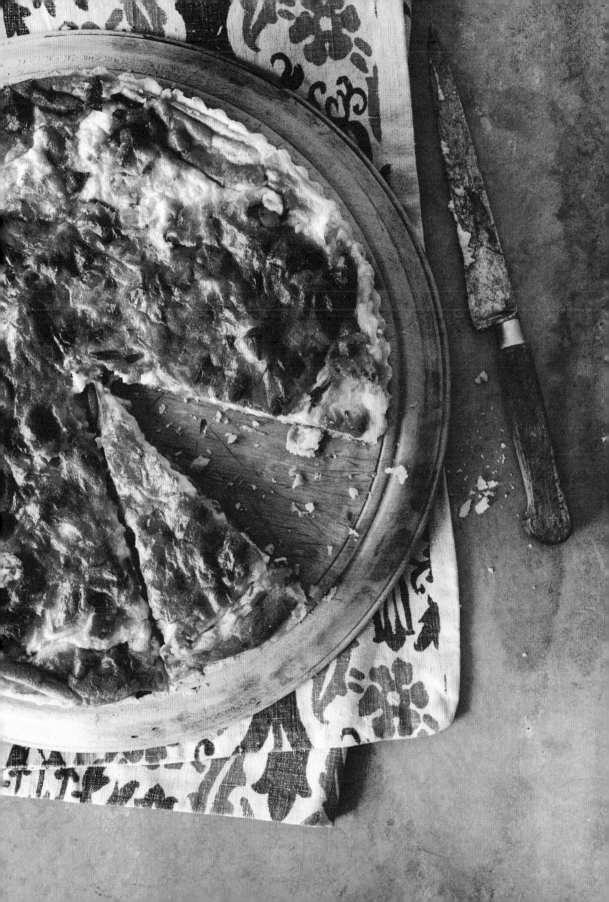

Quiche with crispy back bacon and caramelized onions

For the pastry
275g/2½ cups of white
   spelt flour or plain/all-
   purpose white flour
½ teaspoon of salt
200g/2 sticks of butter
2 eggs, separated
3 tablespoons of water

The pastry of this lovely quiche comes courtesy of Callie Hope-Moreley, and it is a proper French pâte à pâte, (French butter pastry), except I have made it with spelt flour. Oh, for a quiche that puffs up and trembles when it comes out of the oven. I hate those solid lumps of pastry, with solid lumps of egg. I want quivering Cartland heroines in my quiche. As long as they are not pink. I feel like the bacon keeps this sturdy.

Sieve the flour and salt into a food-processor bowl. Cut the butter into small cubes and add it to the flour. Using the pastry blade, whiz up until it resembles fine breadcrumbs. Keeping it on, add the egg yolks and a few spoons of water to mix the dough. Take out the dough and lightly knead into a ball. Wrap in clingfilm and place in the fridge for about half an hour. Preheat the oven to 200°C/180°C fan/Gas 6.

Grease a deep 28cm/11 inch flan dish and roll out the pastry thinly. Line the dish with the pastry, removing any air pockets. Prick the base with a fork and bake blind for 20 minutes.

Whilst the flan base is baking, caramelize the onion. In a heavy-bottomed pan, heat a glug of olive oil and add the onion, stirring and stirring and making sure it is covered in the oil. You want to do this on a low heat as the goal is for the onion to become golden not charred. A heat diffuser can help. This will also take about 20 minutes. Remove the flan and keep to the side. Onion the same. Turn the oven up to 230°C/210°C fan/Gas 8.

In a saucepan, melt the butter and add the flour to make a roux. Add the milk, bit by bit, stirring slowly and continuously until thick and just simmering. Simmer for a few minutes, then add the cheese and stir until melted. Take off the heat and add the bacon, a pinch of mustard powder, salt and pepper and the caramelized onion. In a separate bowl, mix the egg whites until they form stiff peaks, and gently fold them into the lovely roux. Pour it all in to the pastry case and bake for 25 to 30 minutes. Serve immediately.

For the filling

A glug of olive oil

1 large onion, peeled and finely chopped

75g/¾ stick of butter

75g/¾ cup of white spelt flour

570ml/2½ cups of semi-skimmed milk

110g/1 cup of grated Cheddar cheese

225g/8oz of back bacon, grilled and crispy

A pinch of mustard powder

Salt and pepper

... continuously to the wind. Beyond ... ... the new poles with fearful now ... ... of each acted as a sink drawn ... ... may add a strain. Now, ... come teld ... on the poly ... ... a groan, jug ... The orchards are ... Up to the stubble ... already been sown ... ... one, they plough ... ... ed and ridge ... ... fields a regula ... ... help in the hand ... ... sometimes in a ... ... solitary sound ... ... whip. The spot ... to death ... ... of the Belfort ... ... re is plenty of land ... ... land isn't owned by ...

... ful and Berry ...

... quite differently. We'd ... ... to the ready-rich. We'd ... ... yet is aching bones from ... ... the peasants. The boyars ... ... e country. He took the side ... ... e people. As the song ...

... neck ...

"Don't ... ... night hear you and give you ... to the Gove ... ... than you've ever done?"

"Let them do the mo ... tary. All the poor talk about it. There is ... the mayor, maybe the priest, maybe B ... among the barefooted who doesn't complain, who doesn't curse. If ... wrong, we say they are wrong and that's that. The fire smoulders ... ashes. But one day it will break out and we'll see the flames ... Father pokes the fire on the hearth. The fire revives and t ... thinner and turns blue. The curling smoke vanishes up by t ... flames rise yellow first, then red. They lick the bottom of ...

(37)

Winter
Suppers

Winter curry with saffron cinnamon rice

2 tablespoons of safflower
oil

2 onions, peeled and finely
chopped

2 cloves of garlic, peeled
and finely chopped

1 green chilli, deseeded and
finely chopped

1kg/2lb of pumpkin, peeled,
deseeded and roughly
chopped

400g/14oz can of
chickpeas/garbanzo
beans, drained and
rinsed

About 250ml/1½cups of
vegetable stock

400ml/1½cups of coconut
milk

Salt

2 handfuls of mangetout

A handful of fresh
coriander/cilantro

This is sweet and filled with flavour, and you can tailor your garam masala to your own tastes, adjusting as you like. The rice is pretty foolproof, the method taught to me by Peter Begg, a man who knows about food.

In a pestle and mortar, make the garam masala by crushing up and grinding all your dry spices.

In a heavy-bottomed casserole or pan, heat the safflower oil and add the onions, sweating on a low heat until soft and translucent. Add the garlic and stir for another half a minute, taking care not to burn it. Add to this mix the garam masala and chilli and coat the onions with it. Add the pumpkin and the chickpeas/garbanzo beans and then pour over the stock, followed by the coconut milk. Season and simmer for 10 to 15 minutes, add the mangetout, and cook for another 5. Serve with handfuls of coriander/cilantro and the rice.

To make the saffron cinnamon rice, put the rice in a sieve and rinse until the water runs clear. Put the rice in a large saucepan with the water, the butter, cardamom, saffron and cinnamon. Bring to a rolling boil, quickly turn the heat down, put a lid on the saucepan and then leave for 10 minutes. Remove the lid and take it to the table in the saucepan, because it looks like a painting.

For the garam masala
1 teaspoon of cumin seeds
1 teaspoon of mustard
  seeds
½ teaspoon of cloves
1 teaspoon of ground
  turmeric
6 cardamom pods, seeds
  only

For the saffron
cinnamon rice
300g/1½ cups of basmati
  rice
450ml/1¾ cups of water
1 large knob of butter
A couple of cardamom
  pods
A pinch of saffron
2 cinnamon sticks

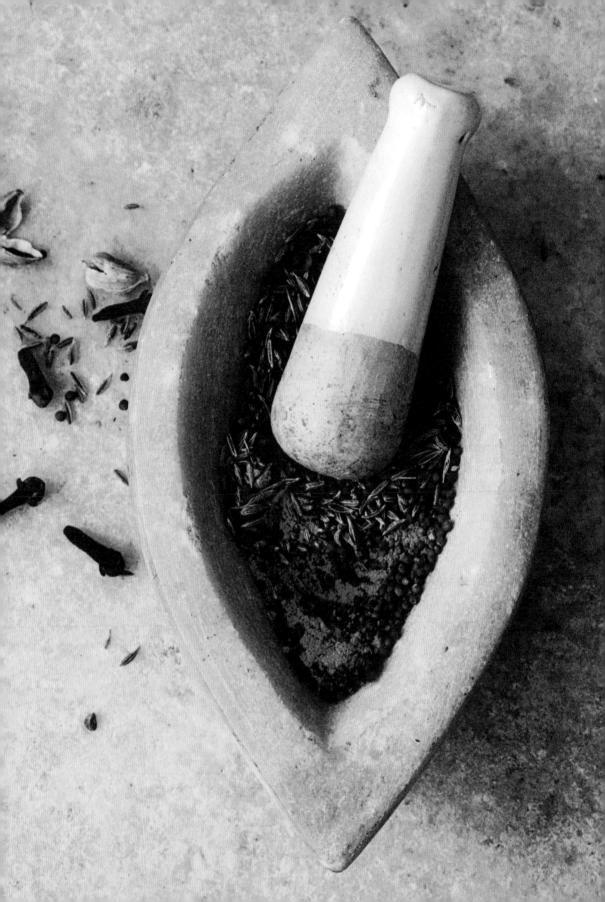

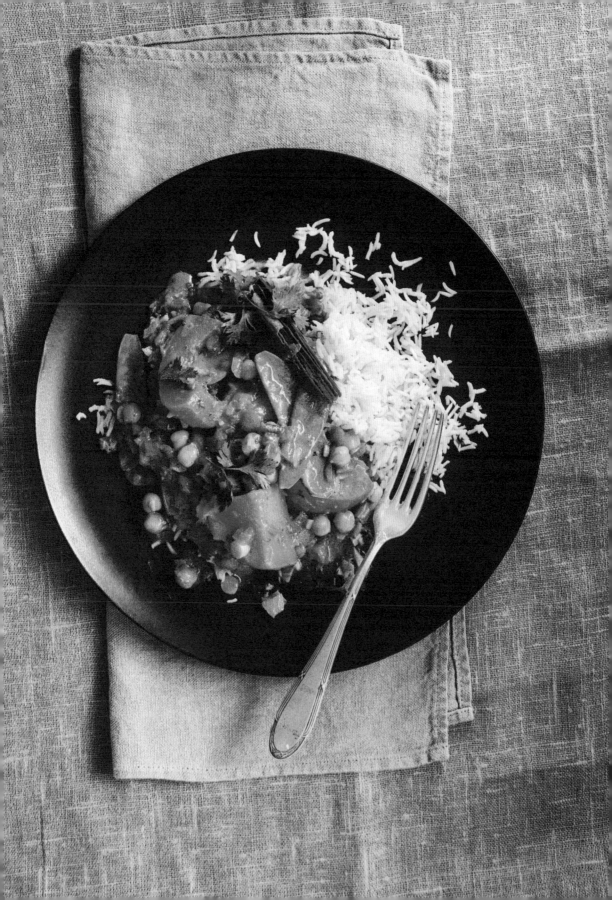

Penne with almond goat's curd parsley pesto

SERVES 6–8

For the pesto
2 cloves of garlic, peeled
Salt and pepper
2 large handfuls of fresh
    parsley
50g/½ cup of blanched
    almonds
200g/1 cup of goat's curd
    or soft goat's cheese
3 tablespoons of olive oil
A squeeze of lemon juice
    or some lemon zest

750g/1½lb of penne pasta

The bottom line is, it's not really pesto in anything but name. You could also spread it on fish before grilling or pan-frying, or puncture a chicken breast and stuff it with it.

In a large pestle and mortar, grind the garlic down with a pinch of sea salt. Add the parsley and again, grind down until you have a coarse green mixture. Add the almonds and keep grinding, and when you have a coarse paste-like consistency, transfer to a larger bowl and add the goat's curd or cheese and olive oil, combining it altogether. Season, giving it a squeeze of lemon or a grating of lemon zest if you feel like it.

Cook the pasta to direction, depending on whether you are using dry or fresh. Reserve a tiny bit of the cooking water when you drain, and add the pesto to the pasta in the pan, making sure it's evenly coated.

Fish fingers with tartare sauce and mushy peas

When the volcanic ash was drifting across Europe, I was travelling with my husband who was working in Australia. Tragically, we got stranded in Sydney for two whole weeks. We took the ferry every day to Manly Beach, swam, read and ate. A lot. This reminds me of one of those Manly Beach afternoons, and having to pretend to everyone back in England that we really minded being stuck.

First make the tartare sauce. In a small mixing bowl, mix the mayonnaise, cornichons, capers and parsley and squeeze in a dash of lemon juice. Add the horseradish and taste, adjusting accordingly. Season.

Make the mushy peas by cooking the frozen peas until al dente, a few minutes, drain them, and then in the saucepan you cooked them in, add them back in and squash them with a potato masher. Add the crème fraîche, olive oil, mint and salt and pepper. Cover and keep to the side.

Cut the fish into finger-sized chunks. Brush a griddle pan with some oil and, when the pan is searing hot, add the fish. Cook for a minute or two on each side. Serve with the mushy peas, the tartare sauce and a lemon wedge.

SERVES 2

300g/10oz of firm-fleshed sustainable white fish, such as coley (ask your fishmonger)
2 tablespoons of olive oil

For the tartare sauce
4 tablespoons of mayonnaise
4 small cornichons, finely chopped
1 large tablespoon of capers
A handful of fresh parsley, finely chopped
A squeeze of lemon juice (keep the other half for wedges)
1 tablespoon of fresh grated horseradish
Salt and pepper

For the peas
150g/1 cup of frozen peas
1 tablespoon of crème fraîche
1 teaspoon of olive oil
1 small handful of fresh chopped mint
Salt and pepper

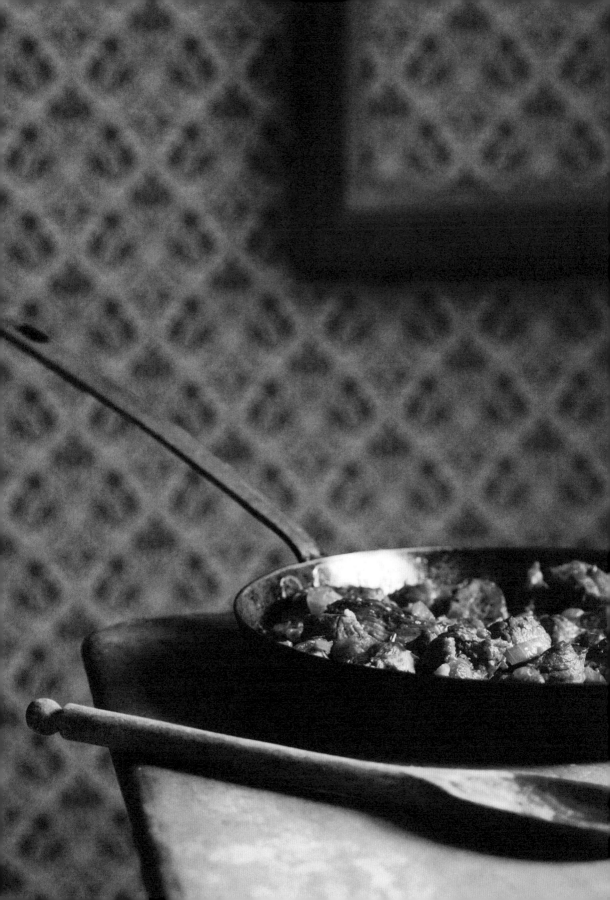

Overnight lamb

Serve it to someone who appreciates a long night.

Brush a casserole lightly with oil and put on a medium to high heat. Brown the lamb in batches if needs be or, if you can, all in one go. This should take 5 minutes or so. When thoroughly brown, set aside on a plate.

On a low heat, sweat the onion and garlic for a few minutes, add the anchovies, stir for a few seconds and then add the stock, followed by the wine. Add the lamb and the rosemary, stir and cook on a low heat for around 30 minutes. Take off the heat and leave the lamb to cool, cover and store overnight in the fridge.

When you are ready for your lamb supper, take the casserole out of the fridge, uncover and put it back on the stove top (you may need to add a little more stock if it has soaked up the juices in the night). Heat on low, adding the mustard, butter and cream and stirring it all through until piping hot.

SERVES 4–6

Olive oil

900g/2lb of lean lamb, cut into small biteable pieces

1 onion, peeled and finely chopped

2 cloves of garlic, peeled and finely chopped

A few anchovies, finely chopped

250ml/1 cup of lamb or chicken stock

185ml/¾ cup of white wine

A handful of fresh chopped rosemary

1 tablespoon of Dijon mustard

1 tablespoon of butter

1 tablespoon of single/light cream

Mushrooms

Vegetable and chicken itame (or an honest stir-fry to the uninitiated!)

In New York I lived near a macrobiotic restaurant that featured a version of this on their menu. It's one of those things to be had when you've been indulging a bit much, that will put you back on the straight and narrow.

Heat the sesame oil in a wok until very hot. Add the chicken strips and cook for a few minutes, then repeat the process with the onion, chilli, cabbage, pepper, mushrooms, carrot and bean sprouts, flash cooking each thing before adding another. Splash with tamari and stir. Mix in the coconut cream and add the lime juice. Serve on rice or some soba noodles.

SERVES 2

1 tablespoon of sesame oil

150g/5oz of skinless and boneless chicken breast, chopped into thin strips

½ an onion, peeled and finely chopped

1 red chilli, deseeded and finely chopped

70g/1 cup of finely shredded green cabbage

1 green (bell) pepper, finely chopped

70g/¾ cup of chopped mushrooms

1 large carrot, coarsely grated

A handful of bean sprouts

2 tablespoons of tamari (wheat-free soy sauce)

1 tablespoon of coconut cream

Juice of 1 lime

Halibut with sorrel sauce and Jerusalem artichoke purée

SERVES 2

2 firm-fleshed sustainable white fish steaks, such as halibut (ask your fishmonger)
Salt and pepper
Olive oil
Lemon

For the Jerusalem artichoke purée
250g/9oz of Jerusalem artichokes
300ml/1¼ cups of milk
A knob of butter
Salt and pepper

For the sauce
1 small bunch of sorrel
A handful of fresh tarragon
2 large tablespoons of crème fraîche
1 tablespoon of olive oil
Juice of ½ a lemon
Salt and pepper

Halibut is a fish to treat with care and have rarely as, like cod, it is being overfished. It is meaty and wonderful, particularly good served with something soft, à la the artichoke purée or champ.

Preheat the oven to 200°C/180°C fan/Gas 6. Peel the Jerusalem artichokes, place in a pan and pour the milk over them. Cook them on a low heat until tender, about 10 to 15 minutes. Drain, saving a little bit of the milk, and put in the blender with a knob of butter and the reserved milk. Season and keep warm to one side.

Wash and dry the fish and season, brushing with a little olive oil. Heat a griddle pan and, when searing hot, place the fish in it, skin side down. Cook for a few minutes, and then turn and place in the hot oven for 10 minutes.

While the fish is cooking, blanch the sorrel in a pan of boiling water for no more than 30 seconds. Quickly submerge into iced water, then squeeze all the water out. Chop the sorrel finely along with the tarragon and, in a small bowl, mix it in with the crème fraîche, the olive oil, the lemon juice and salt and pepper.

Put the Jerusalem artichoke on a plate, place the fish on top of it, and serve with a generous dollop of sauce.

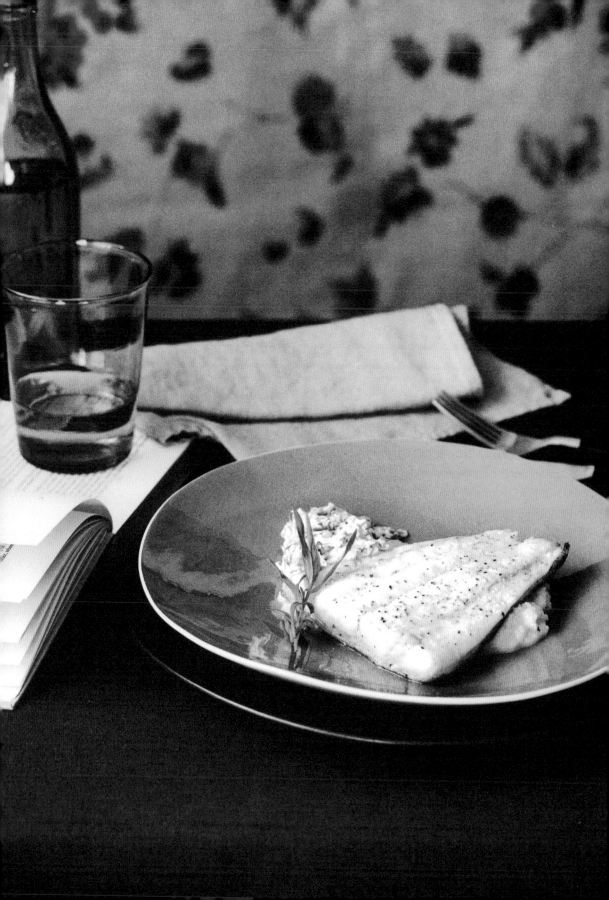

The second Mor Mor's chicken

My Mor Mor was not Norwegian at all. She was born Patsy Louise in Packard, Kentucky, in what she called a 'hillbilly' coal mining camp. When she married my grandfather, she decided that she liked the name Mor Mor, and that when she was a grandmother, she would take it as her own. And she did.

She had a laugh that traversed years of cigarettes and jokes, and rang out like a deep, dirty well.

Her chicken is the stuff of fable amongst my aunts, and when I'd talk to them about recipes, they would always bang on about Mor Mor's chicken from their childhood. The problem was, neither of them could really remember what was in it, they just remembered the ultimate result being delicious. They muttered about mushrooms, they muttered about tarragon.

'Ring Mor Mor!' They urged me.

'Mor Mor, what was in your chicken?' I asked Mor Mor, who was sipping her nightly martini in New York.

'Christ, I don't know baby. Chicken?' Mor Mor said.

Mor Mor, coaxed and prodded, didn't remember. She thought it may have something to do with Campbell's Soup, but I'm not so sure, because it sounded disgusting. I resolved that maybe they just all had different taste in the seventies.

She had many incarnations and her name and its changes embodied them. She became Patricia when Broadway beckoned in the mid 1940s. She would always honour her roots, and she could conjure a country twang in a heartbeat with the throaty voice that would be her lifelong moniker. Her down-home ways and grit were one of the many things that endeared her to Gary Cooper, with whom she co-starred in *The Fountainhead* in 1949. They embarked on a love affair that would devastate both of them. She met my grandfather on the rebound from Cooper in 1951, at a dinner party thrown by Lillian Hellman. He totally ignored her, although he sat next to her, but to her surprise he called her the next morning to ask her out for dinner. She told him she was busy, but he persisted, and after a while she said, recalling it for me years later, she simply ran out of excuses.

They married in New York in 1953, and were to have five children together. Their son Theo was in his baby carriage in New York in 1960 when he was hit by a taxi running a red light. He suffered brain damage that eventually took the family home to their farmhouse in England. Two years later, their seven-year-old daughter Olivia contracted measles encephalitis and died. It is astonishing to look back on Patricia's numerous awards at this time (including an Oscar for best actress in *Hud* in 1963) with the knowledge that her domestic life was dissolving around her. In 1965, pregnant with her fifth child, Lucy, Patricia suffered three cerebral aneurysms, which left her in a coma for nearly a month. When she came round she was left without language or memory, paralyzed on her right side. Her rehabilitation is the stuff of legend, and the courage that she displayed throughout the long, dark days of recovery, undeniable. She learnt to walk and talk, read and write, all over again, with the support of her husband and neighbours, a martini and cigarette never far from reach. She was nominated for another Academy Award in 1968, for her work in *The Subject Was Roses*. Her homecoming speech, as it were, brought her peers to their feet in a standing ovation, as those whisky chords tumbled over each other to proclaim, 'I am so happy to be alive. Alive, alive-O.'

Her fervency was real. Her life was one rich with beauty and unbearable injustice. Throughout it all, she retained a stellar sense of humour, faith and a heart big enough to carry our entire family. She delighted in the simple; the depth of a sunflower, a doggy bag, a loud curse word or filthy story. In the dearth of her short-term memory, one was 'Darling', 'Divine One' or 'Beauty', and anyone who has been so addressed by her would know the honour that it carried. She was regal in every inch of her being, even in the face of the cancer that ravaged her. She told my aunt Ophelia that she was 'a little offended' she had cancer, and why shouldn't she be? She had been so close to death in her life, danced neatly away from him, and here he was again, darkening her door.

Our beloved Mor Mor died in August 2010 in her own bed, surrounded by her family. She told me she'd be gone before my baby was born, and she was right. The night before, she had dinner with her kids, kissed them each, raised a glass, and told them she'd had 'A lovely time'.

The secret of her mysterious chicken died with her. The following is my imagined Mor Mor's chicken, in tribute to all of her gutsy glory, beauty and tenacity. If it was to be eaten and enjoyed Mor Mor style, it would involve copious amounts of corn bread, white wine and some matinée-idol handsome men to eat it with.

Eat it with the people you love the most, and don't waste it on the dull.

In a large casserole, heat a tablespoon of oil and add the chicken pieces to brown. Turn the pieces after a few minutes to make sure they are evenly coloured. When all are brown, add the onion, garlic, bay leaves, herbes de Provence and chicken stock and cook on a low to medium heat for about 10 to 15 minutes. To test doneness, take a piece of chicken out and pierce, making sure the juices run clear. If they don't, put back and cook for another 5 minutes. When the chicken has cooked, take it carefully out of the casserole and keep to one side.

Leaving the stocky juices, take the onion and garlic out of the casserole and throw them in the compost or in the bin. Reduce the stock by half, by boiling it up and bringing it back down again. Add the wine and season. Add the mushrooms and cook for 5 minutes, and then add the peas and cook for another 3 or 4. Lastly, gently stir in the cream, and then the herbs. Put the chicken back in the casserole, season and take to the table. Delicious with mashed potatoes.

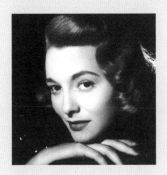

SERVES 4

1 tablespoon of olive oil
4 skinless and boneless chicken breasts, chopped into bite-sized pieces
1 onion, peeled but whole
1 bulb of garlic, cut in half
2 bay leaves
A pinch of herbes de Provence
1.2 litres/5 cups of chicken stock (preferably fresh free-range chicken stock)
125ml/½ cup of white wine
A large pinch of salt
A pinch of pepper
250g/3 cups of wild mushrooms
250g/1½ cups of frozen peas
300ml/1¼ cups of double/heavy cream
A handful each of fresh parsley, chervil and tarragon, finely chopped

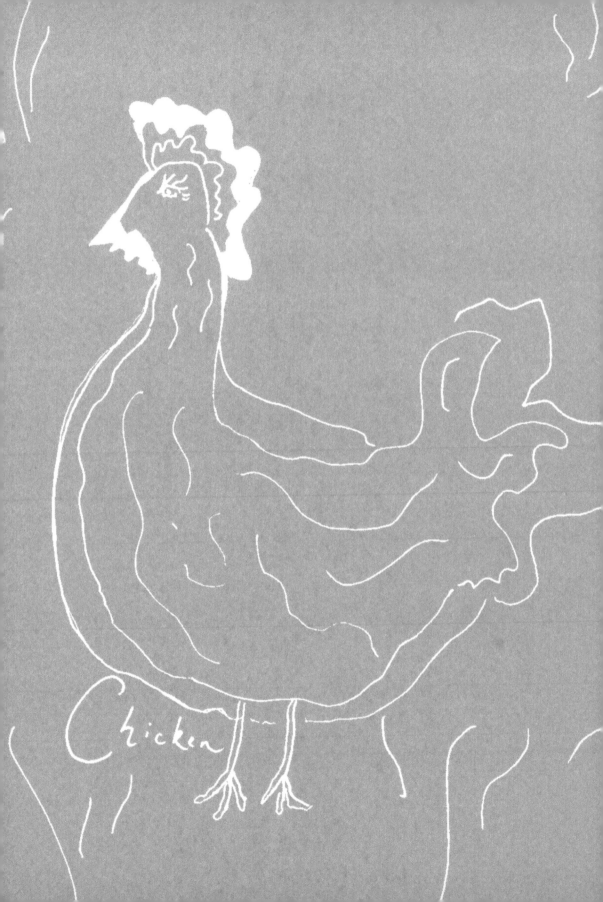

Chicken

Spring

BREAKFASTS
Rhubarb rice pudding
Courgette/zucchini hotcakes
Halloumi croque madame with black olives
Apple and raspberry cereal
Spicy aubergine/eggplant and tomato with poached eggs
Avocado nut milk smoothie
Rye cracker breads with horseradish and smoked trout pâté

LUNCHES
Asparagus with hard-boiled eggs, Parmesan and lemon
Bruschetta with artichoke purée
Hot smoked salmon tacos
Butter lettuce, lobster and crayfish/crawfish salad
Crespou
Pea, pesto and rocket/arugula soup
Potato pancakes with smoked salmon and a cucumber and dill salad

SUPPERS
Macky Boy's mackerel with baby spinach and horseradish dressing
Coconut and crab rice with lime and coriander/cilantro
Pollack with Indian spices and yoghurt lime dressing
Lemon lentil soup
Paella
Chicken Kiev
The Sheriff's marinated lamb

I couldn't sleep, and I started to think about the rhubarb poking its sleepy head out in the garden.

In her famous book of household management, the Victorian domestic advisor, Isabella Beeton, suggests rhubarb only in the form of an economical jam for making in the months of February to April. I am suggesting it as a rice pudding, or on its own, boiled up with a bit of sugar, because it seems such a travesty in the spring not to celebrate rhubarb then and there. If you have an abundance, of course, jam is the sensible way of prolonging the feast.

I am a huge devotee of Mrs Beeton, the somewhat faceless author of a cookbook that has sold in the millions, and continues to be reprinted and revised, year after year. She styled herself as the original domestic goddess, but her true talent was in entrepreneurship and marketing. Her recipes do little for me, and are pretty unappealing to a modern palate, but I love her unconventional story and spirit. Today, she'd be a multimillionaire. She saw a gap in the market, in the form of the newly growing middle classes, who were looking for a calm, authoritative voice on everything from roasting meat to finding a wet nurse if you were having trouble breastfeeding. The tone she projects in her book is one of matronly competence, but in reality, she was a twenty-three-year-old fashion journalist and editor, a newlywed, more comfortable at an office desk than the oven. She was however, a keen and adept baker. Brought up in Cheapside, then Epsom, she taps into the subconscious of her urban Victorian reader, suspicious of food adulteration and intensive farming, a reader who yearns at moments for the simple rural idyll that precedes them, their steam trains, servants and mills. In her syllabub recipe, Mrs Beeton invites you to, 'Milk directly into the bowl,' as though available cows udders are two a penny in the borough of Bow. What she is getting at remains timeless; the thirst for perfection sought through domestic bibles. We can learn much about history and the habits and dreams of a nation through its old cookbooks. There is Eliza Acton, a marvellous food writer who came before Mrs Beeton (indeed Mrs B shamelessly plagiarized quite a few of her recipes); Ambrose Heath (introduced to me by Peter Begg, a fountain of food knowledge), a waspishly funny columnist for *The Times* and *Guardian* who published books in the 1930s; Alice B. Toklas, wry lover of Gertrude Stein and heavenly food writer and cook; M.F.K. Fisher, author of novels and studies of food, including the brilliant *Serve it Forth*; Jane Grigson, whose books on vegetables are modern-day classics, Elizabeth David, who brought French Provençal cooking to the masses. These are six food writers who I'm thinking of on the spur of the moment, in amidst thoughts of rhubarb and not sleeping. There are myriad others to add to this list, both living and dead. Do explore them if you don't already know them, and you love reading about food, because you will be richly rewarded.

We are now in the season of change; embrace it with abandon! The garden is abundant with possibility; spinach and lettuce are in season, tender and the perfect green foil for the meat you serve them with.

Spring is a time of firsts, warm with romance, bloom and promise. If you can't be bothered with cooking, make like the French on the first of May and find some lily of the valley, keeping your table as sweet as the changing landscape.

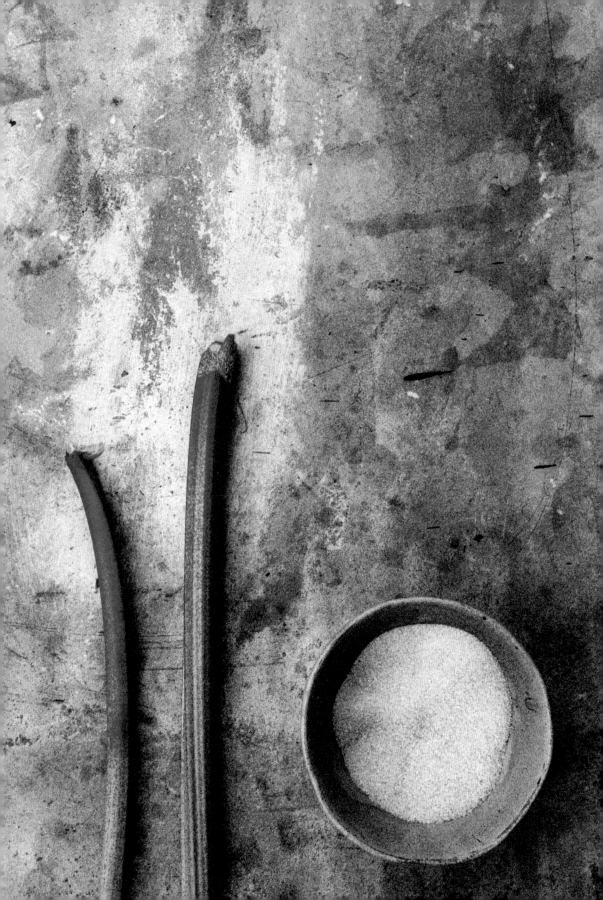

Spring Breakfasts

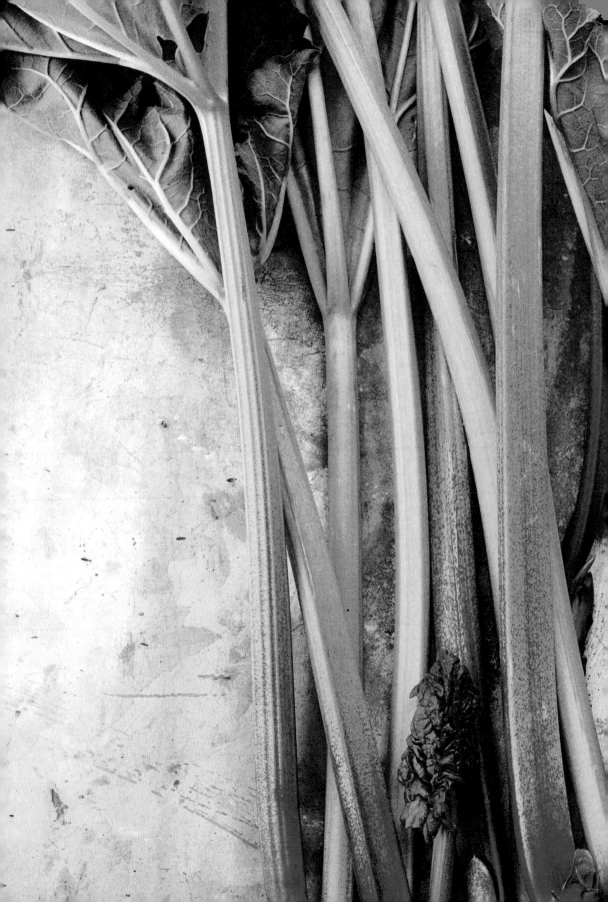

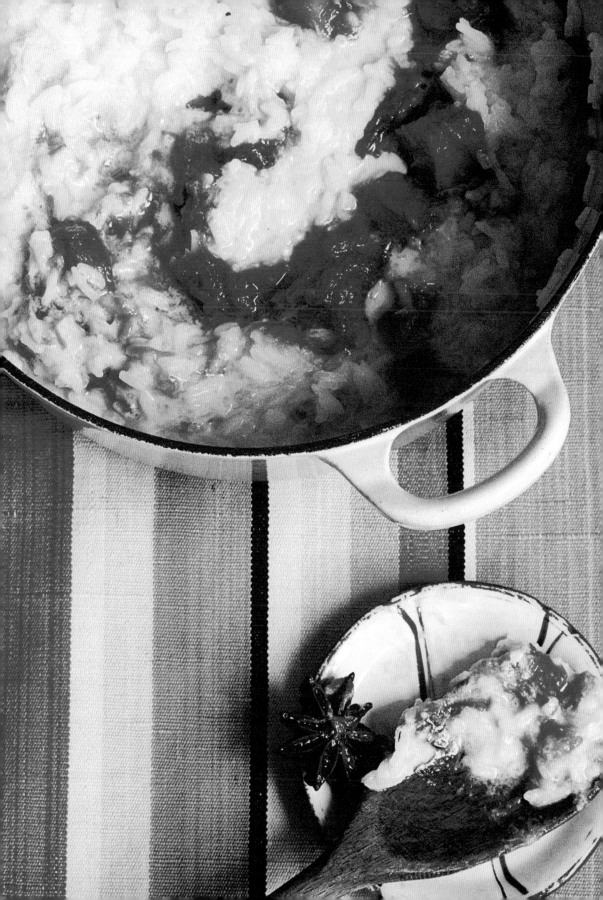

Rhubarb rice pudding

SERVES 2

1 litre/4 cups of milk

150g/¾ cup of basmati rice

1 cinnamon stick

80g/¼ cup of agave syrup
   or honey

1 teaspoon of orange
   flower water

For the rhubarb

350g/12oz of rhubarb, cut
   into 2.5cm/1 inch lengths

125ml/½ cup of water

1 star anise

1 teaspoon of rosewater

2 tablespoons of agave
   syrup or honey

I used to pick rhubarb in my granny Gee-Gee's garden when I was about seven, with a bowl of sugar clutched in my fat little hand. The trick was to lick the rhubarb, dip it in the sugar, and crunch away. I would always do it to excess, which was a sure-fire way to aching guts, and Gee-Gee clucking over me with some milk of magnesia. Prepared this way, you have all the joy without the pain, and if you have access to a bumper crop, follow Mrs Beeton's example and make some jam.

First make the rice pudding. Pour the milk and rice into a medium-sized saucepan, add the cinnamon stick, bring to the boil, and then simmer on a very low heat, stirring frequently, for around 30 minutes. At this point, stir in the agave or honey and the orange flower water and cook for another 5 to 10 minutes, adding more milk if it starts looking dry.

In a separate heavy-bottomed pan, place the rhubarb, water, star anise, rosewater and agave or honey. Bring to the boil and simmer on low for about 10 minutes, turning once or twice, until you have a lovely tender pink softness. Plate the rice pudding and swirl the rhubarb through.

Courgette/zucchini hotcakes

Celebrating the green of spring, the gold of first sun and the all-round brilliance that is cheese. You can also serve these for tea with a bit of butter.

Preheat the oven to about 190°C/170°C fan/Gas 5 and grease eight holes of a large capacity muffin tray/trays.

I stick all of this in the KitchenAid – but you can do it in a mixing bowl as easily. Start with the dry ingredients, sifting in the flour and baking powder. Slowly add the egg, oil and milk, whisking all the while. Add the courgette/zucchini, the cheese and the thyme and season to taste. Pour into the prepared trays and bake for around 20 minutes or until golden.

MAKES 8

230g/2 cups of spelt flour
1 teaspoon of baking
    powder
1 egg
60ml/¼ cup of olive oil
170ml/⅔ cup of milk
1 courgette/zucchini,
    coarsely grated
100g/1 cup of grated
    Parmesan
1 tablespoon of fresh
    chopped thyme
Salt and pepper

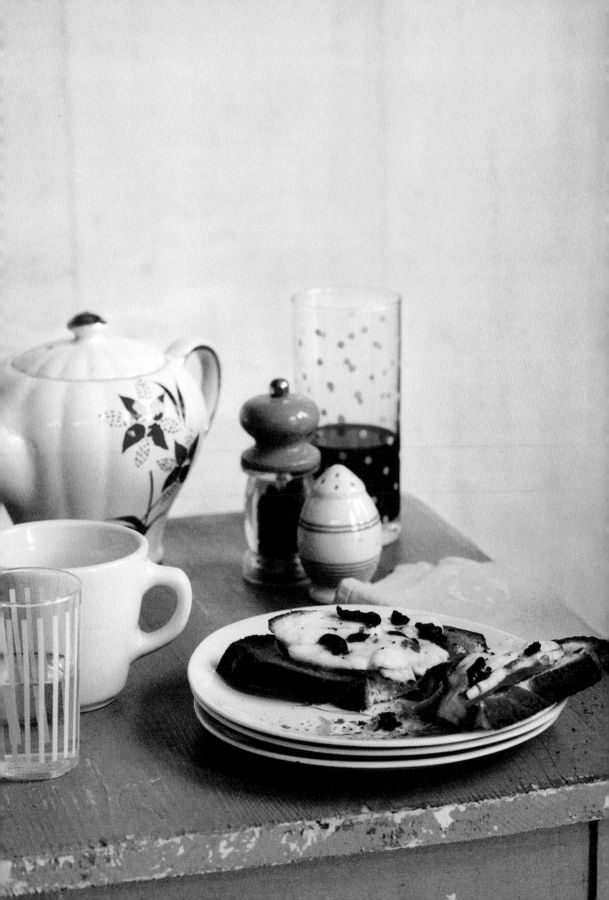

Halloumi croque madame with black olives

After a very late concert in Paris, from which we spilled out into torrential rain, my husband and I found ourselves in one of those cafés you dream about. Safe from the downpour, we were greeted with deep glasses of red wine and the classic sandwich – oozing slabs of Gruyère atop Poilâne bread, his with ham, mine with an egg. When we were back home, I tried to do the same with some halloumi, which was what I happened to have in the fridge. It wouldn't thrill the French, but it was pretty bloody marvellous all the same. Poilâne bread is so named after the French baker, Lionel Poilâne, and it is made from sourdough and stoneground flours, spelt flour, and naturally fermented and baked in a traditional wood fired oven. A rustic sourdough will do in place of it.

Preheat the grill to High. Lightly toast the bread, butter it, and cover evenly with one layer of ham and then the halloumi. Chop the olives and press them into the halloumi, as much as you can. Put them under the piping hot grill for 4 minutes or so, or until the cheese is golden and bubbling.

MAKES 2

2 slices of challah bread or, my favourite, Poilâne
A knob of butter
2 slices of Serrano ham
Enough halloumi to generously cover (about 100g/3½oz)
6 pitted black olives

Apple and raspberry cereal

SERVES 2

200g/2 cups of porridge
  oats
250ml/1 cup of water
2 apples – Russets work
  well here
A handful of raspberries
Some milk or apple juice,
  to moisten
A small spoon of runny
  honey

This is a bit of a cheat because raspberries really start rearing their heads in early summer, May/June. The crows in my garden would attest to this fact as they are a sucker for berries. However, you can substitute another fruit here, maybe some rhubarb? I love a good Bircher muesli-ish cereal; they are simple as anything, and very virtuous.

The night before, put the porridge in a bowl and pour the water on top. Grate the apple onto the oats and add the raspberries. Refrigerate overnight and in the morning moisten with some milk or apple juice. Swirl in the honey and eat.

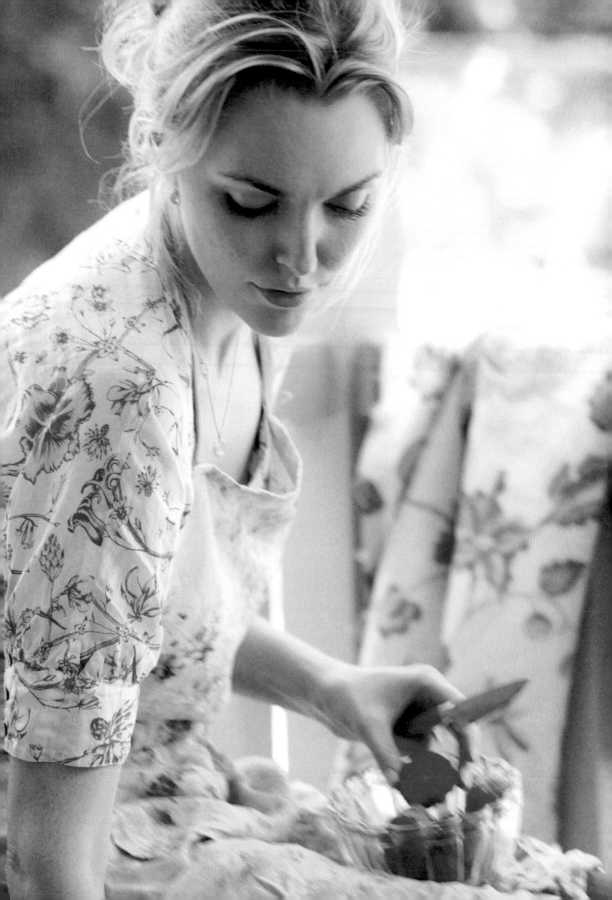

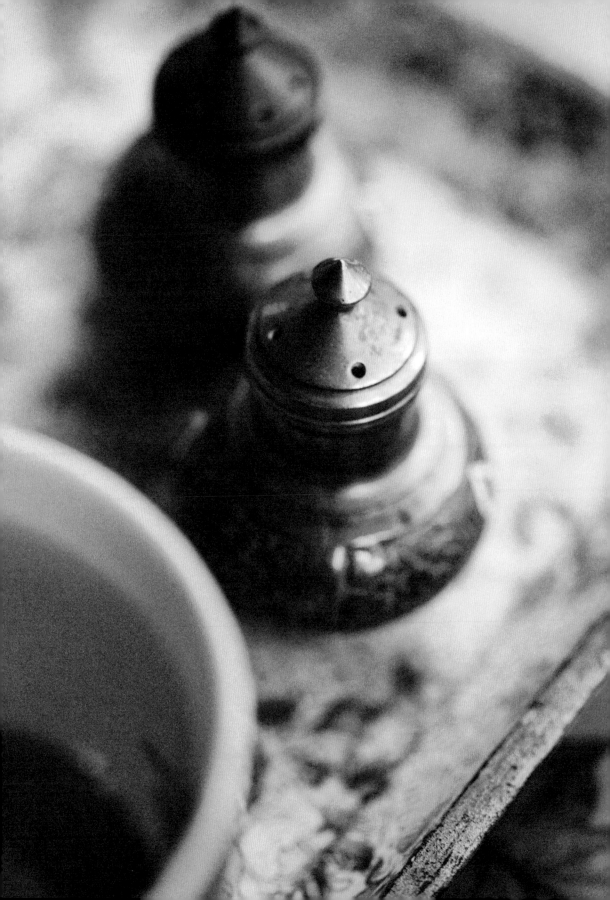

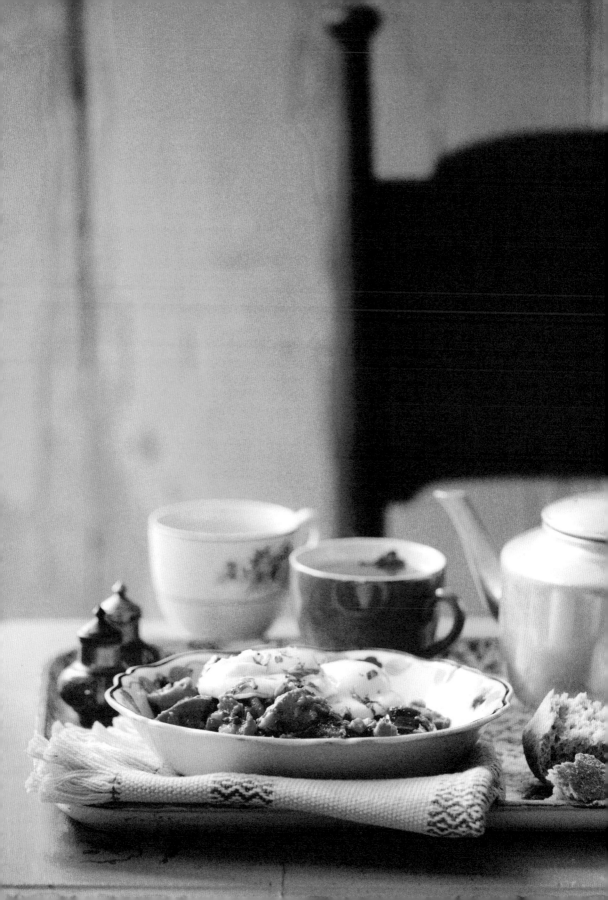

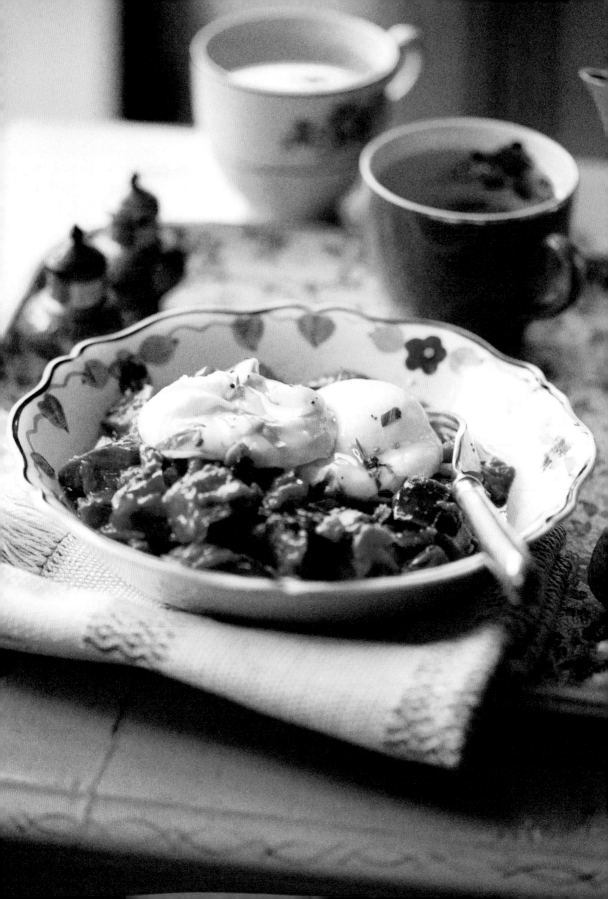

Spicy aubergine/eggplant and tomato with poached eggs

This was another dinner thing, served at a party on a warm spring night with some couscous. Like so often with soups and stews that have spent a night in the fridge, they are even better re-imagined the following morning. Maybe it was just the hangover, but I looked at this and thought, 'Hmm, I bet that would be good with some eggs on top.' It was, and remains to be, even stone cold sober.

Cut the aubergine/eggplant into bite-sized chunks, and soak for about 20 minutes in a bowl of cold water with a few large pinches of salt. Drain and rinse and pat dry.

In a heavy-bottomed pan, heat a tablespoon of oil, add the garlic and onion, and cook for a few minutes until softened. Add the aubergine/eggplant with the rest of the oil, making sure it is thoroughly coated, then add the paprika and cook on a very low heat, covered, for about half an hour, turning occasionally. Add the tomatoes, the tahini and the brown sugar and cook for another 10 minutes, mixing it all through. Taste and season accordingly. Keep warm to the side.

Poach the eggs in a pan of gently boiling water (a splash of white wine vinegar should stop them separating). You should poach the eggs for about 3 minutes if you want them soft in the middle (5 if you want them stern and unyielding).

At the last moment, add the lemon juice and parsley to the aubergine/eggplant mixture. Plate in shallow bowls and place the poached eggs on top, with perhaps a hunk of sourdough to sop up the juices.

SERVES 2

1 large aubergine/eggplant
Salt and pepper
2 tablespoons of olive oil
1 clove of garlic, peeled and finely chopped
1 onion, peeled and finely chopped
½ teaspoon of smoked paprika
250g/1 cup of tomatoes, chopped
1 teaspoon of tahini
1 teaspoon of brown sugar
A splash of white wine vinegar
4 eggs
1 tablespoon of lemon juice
A handful of fresh chopped parsley

Avocado nut milk smoothie

SERVES 1

½ a ripe avocado

A small handful of blanched almonds

A few chunks of frozen banana

250ml/1 cup of cold water or soy milk

A small spoonful of agave syrup or honey

When I went on a strange raw food diet, this sort of smoothie was a prominent feature. So was my bum after months of eating avocado and nuts in spades! In a BALANCED way, this is super good for you, and deeply moreish. Just don't start having four under the illusion that they are thinning in any way.

Throw all of it in the blender and purée until smooth.

Rye cracker breads with horseradish and smoked trout pâté

The credit here goes to the very talented Danish chef and food writer, Trina Hahnemann. I just tinkered with it, and give it to you with huge thanks to her. This is also wonderful as a canapé or starter.

For the pâté, put all of these ingredients in the blender and whiz until smooth. Season to taste. Refrigerate for a few hours. For the rye breads, dissolve the yeast in the warm water in a mixing bowl (or in a KitchenAid with the bread hook), then add the salt, aniseed, honey and oil and mix well. Add the rye flour, oats and half the wheat flour and mix for 5 minutes. Sprinkle the rest of the wheat flour over the dough and leave it to rise for 15 minutes.

Preheat the oven to 200°C/180°C fan/Gas 6 and line a baking sheet with baking/parchment paper. Knead the dough on a floured work surface, then divide it into ten equal pieces and roll each one into a very thin disc. Lay the flatbreads on the baking/parchment paper and bake for 5 to 8 minutes until crisp. Serve the pâté smeared on the crackers.

SERVES 4

For the pâté
2 fillets of smoked trout
50g/¼ cup of soft cream cheese
A pinch of cayenne pepper
Lemon juice, to taste
A tablespoon or so of fresh grated horseradish
1 tablespoon of light olive oil
Salt and pepper

For the rye cracker breads
3 tablespoons of fresh yeast
500ml/2 cups of warm water
1 teaspoon of salt
2 teaspoons of aniseed
1 teaspoon of honey
100ml/scant ½ cup of sunflower oil
200g/2 cups of rye flour
200g/2 cups of rolled oats
250g/1⅔ cups of wholemeal/whole wheat flour

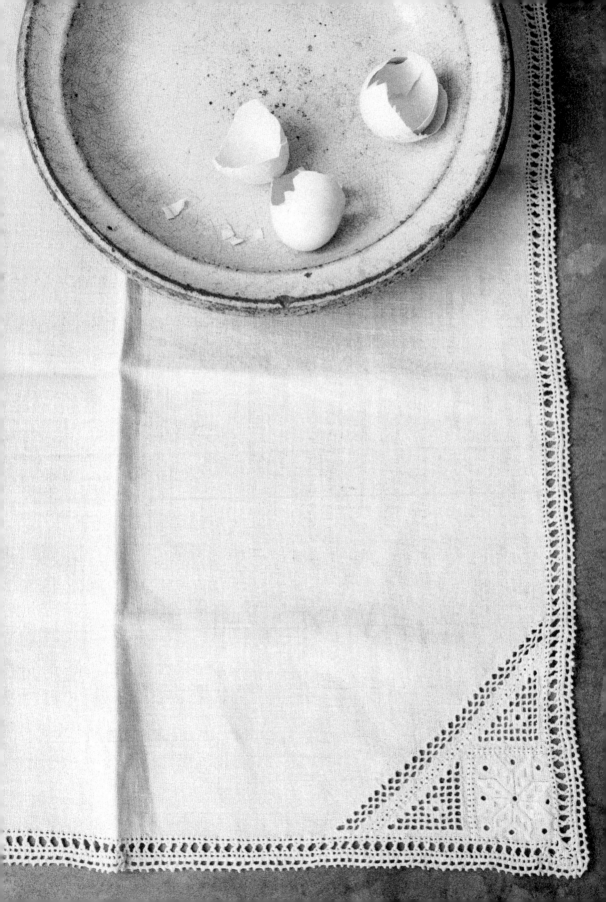

Spring Lunches

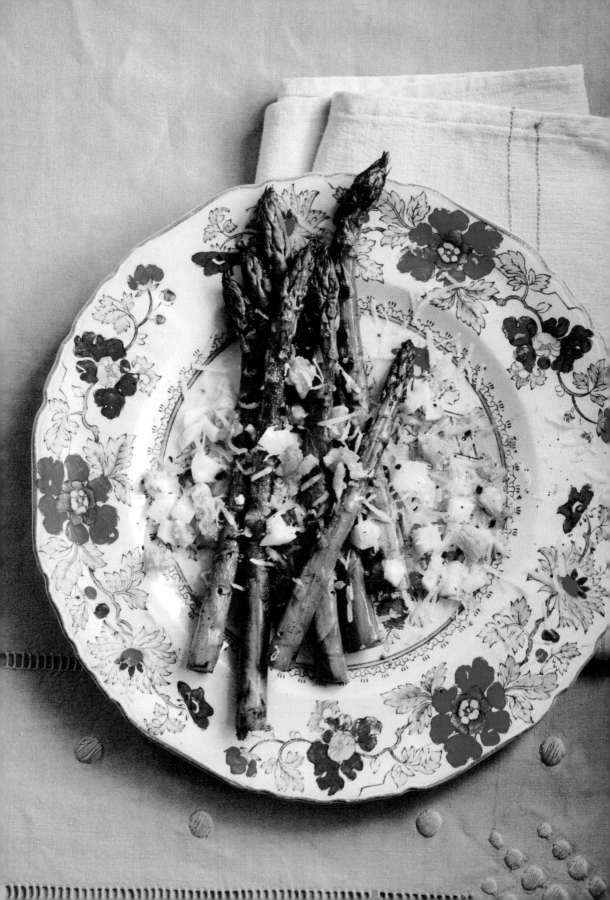

Asparagus with hard-boiled eggs, Parmesan and lemon

There is something totally magical about the lunches of late spring. The first ceremonial throwing open of the windows, or if you have a garden, venturing a picnic with a layer of thermals.

Asparagus will forever remind me of late spring and early summer in England. I made it last for my girlfriend Emma when she was eight months pregnant and we sat and ate it on her roof. Don't serve it for a romantic lunch – you shouldn't need me to tell you why. And why, oh why, do they ever serve asparagus on airplanes?! I would have this alongside a soup to keep you warm.

Heat a griddle pan over a very high heat. Remove the tough ends from the asparagus and cook for about 5 minutes on each side, until browning on the outside and soft within.

While this is cooking, boil the eggs; about 4 or 5 minutes if you want them still slightly runny inside. Plunge them into cold water and peel, chopping finely.

Plate the asparagus, pouring over the olive oil, Parmesan, the lemon juice and the zest. Season and sprinkle the hard-boiled eggs on top.

SERVES 2

A bunch of asparagus, say
 6 per person
2 eggs
2 tablespoons of olive oil
25g/¼ cup of grated
 Parmesan
Juice and grated zest of
 ½ a lemon
Salt and pepper

Bruschetta with artichoke purée

2 medium-sized artichokes

3 tablespoons of olive oil

1 clove of garlic, peeled and
   finely chopped

Juice and grated zest of
   1 lemon

Salt and pepper

2 thick slices of sourdough
   bread

A small handful of fresh
   torn basil

These are great things to serve if you have a lot of people for lunch or dinner before the main course is ready, or if you are trying to be grown up and have people over for 'drinks'. I've never accomplished this. It's either lunch or dinner.

Break off the artichoke stalks and snap or cut off all the leaves. Spoon out the wispy choke and discard. Cut the artichoke hearts in quarters. Heat the olive oil in a medium-sized frying pan and sweat the garlic. Add the artichokes and a teacup full of water and cook on low for about 30 minutes.

When softened, transfer the artichokes to the blender, add the lemon juice, zest and a splash more olive oil and purée, then season to taste. Heat a griddle pan until it's searing, put the sourdough in and cook for a minute or two on each side.

Serve spread with the artichoke purée and the torn basil on top.

Hot smoked salmon tacos

Some dear friends, now Mr and Mrs Collins (not Joan or Phil!) got married last year in a magical place called Cayucos in California. A sleepy seaside town, it held two spectacular gastronomic weapons: salted brown butter cookies, which would fell a stony-hearted puritan, and tacos, which we ate the day after the wedding at Ruddell's Smokehouse, a tiny wooden shed by the water. The tacos exploded with flavour – enigmatic and intense – and that first bite will live with me until I'm grey and ancient. Here they are for your delectation. The cookies I haven't quite figured out yet, but you can imagine them in the interim.

Mix the mayonnaise and sour cream together in a large mixing bowl and add the chilli, cumin, lemon juice and coriander/cilantro. Flake in the hot smoked salmon and season to taste. Put the mixture into the warmed taco shells and top with the shredded cabbage, tomatoes and a wedge of lime.

SERVES 6 HUNGRY PEOPLE

125g/½ cup of mayonnaise
125g/½ cup of sour cream
1 tablespoon of dried red
    chilli flakes
1 tablespoon of ground
    cumin
2 tablespoons of lemon
    juice
A big handful of
    fresh chopped
    coriander/cilantro
450g/1lb of hot smoked
    salmon or any
    smoked fish
Salt and pepper
6 taco shells warmed
A handful of shredded red
    cabbage
2 tomatoes, finely chopped
2 limes, to be cut in
    wedges

Butter lettuce, lobster and crayfish/ crawfish salad

SERVES 4

1 butter lettuce

235g/1½ cups of fresh or frozen peas

450g/1lb of cooked lobster meat

250g/9oz of cooked crayfish/crawfish or prawns/shrimp

1 large avocado (with no brown bits please)

A handful of pea shoots

For the dressing

1 tablespoon of white wine vinegar

½ teaspoon of Dijon mustard

½ teaspoon of agave syrup or caster/superfine sugar

5 tablespoons of light olive oil

3 tablespoons of sour cream, thinned with the juice of 1 lemon

A handful of fresh chopped tarragon and/or chervil

Salt and pepper

Everything about this just works. Sweet, creamy and hearty, it would work as a stand-alone lunch on a warm day. You could also make it as a starter for a dinner party. It makes me think of Oslo, a place that I love and that I visited for the first time only two years ago, which is odd because half of my family hails from there. I could live in the lovely clean airport, where you can get open-faced rye sandwiches galore, piled high with crayfish and mayonnaise. Yum. You can also use the dressing on a cold barbecued piece of chicken.

To make the dressing, put the vinegar, mustard and agave or sugar in a mixing bowl and stir in the olive oil. When amalgamated, add the sour cream, lemon and herbs. Season to taste. Wash the butter lettuce, dry and tear the leaves off carefully. I would serve this in one big low salad bowl so you can admire the beauty of it. Cook the peas very briefly in boiling salted water, literally a minute or two, so they're still tender. Drain them and leave to cool.

Chop the lobster meat into rounds and add this and the crayfish/crawfish to the salad. Pour on the peas. Just before you serve, chop the avocado into half moons and add to the salad bowl. Dress it and add the pea shoots.

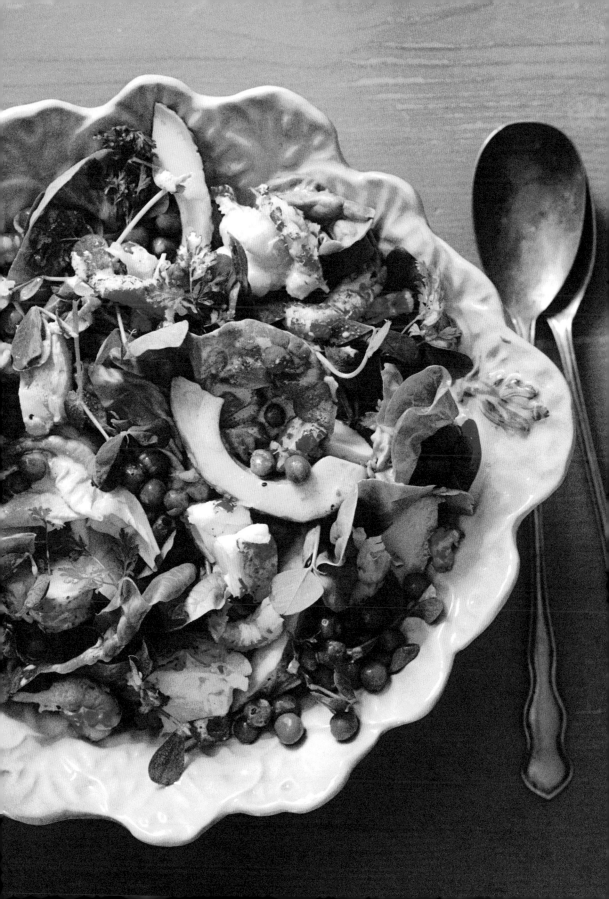

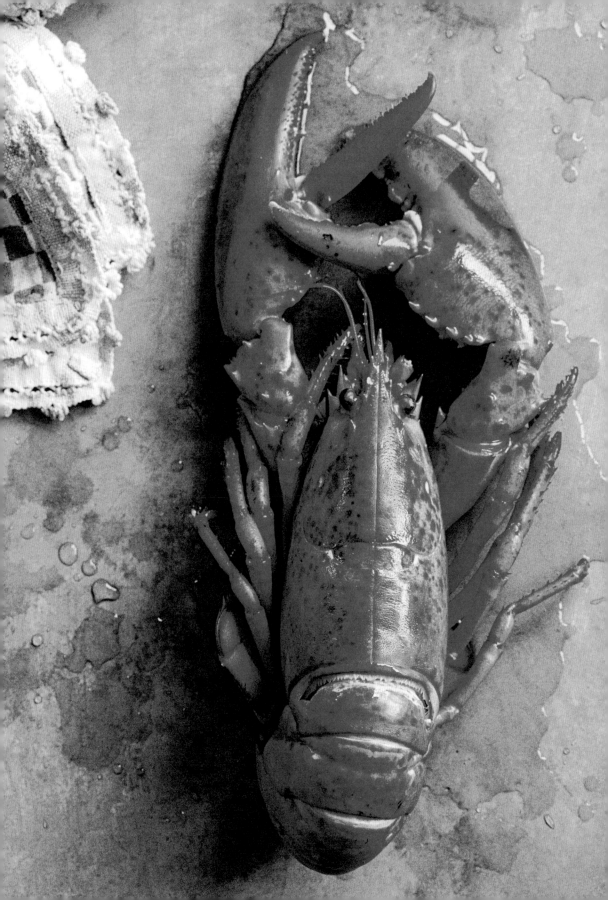

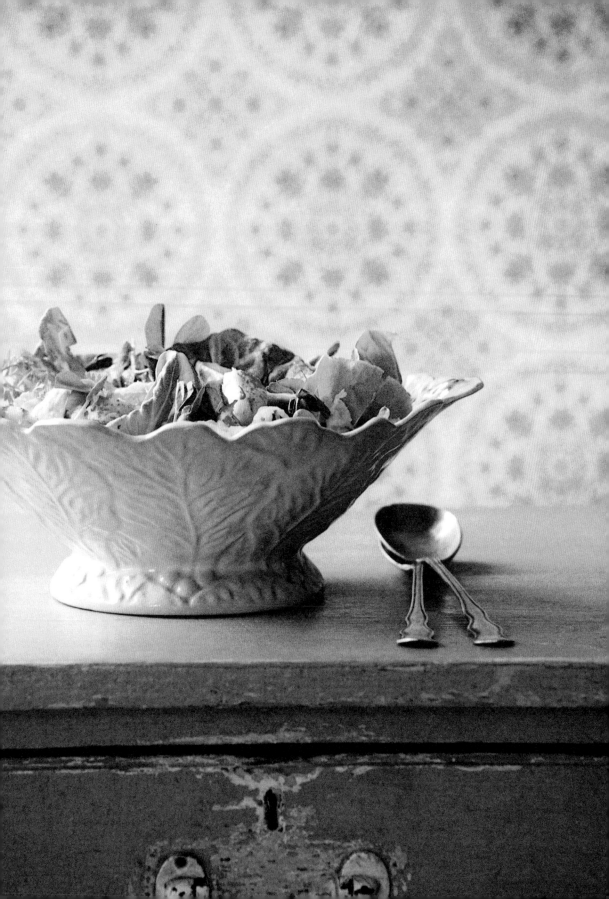

Crespou

SERVES 6

For the yellow omelette

5 eggs

1 tablespoon of
single/light cream

Salt and pepper

Olive oil

1 small onion, peeled and
finely chopped

A few threads of saffron,
soaked in a little hot
cream or water

For the green omelette

5 eggs

Salt and pepper

Olive oil

A handful of baby spinach

3 tablespoons of fresh
chopped tarragon

1 tablespoon of fresh
chopped parsley

25g/¼ cup of grated
Parmesan

For the red omelette

5 eggs

Salt and pepper

Olive oil

8 cherry tomatoes,
quartered

25g/¼ cup of crumbled
goat's cheese

Fresh chopped soft herbs,
to garnish

You can be creative with a Crespou and mix and match the fillings – the ones I've picked are the things I happened to have to hand. Crespou is a Provençal omelette cake in essence, with each layer offering a different colour and flavour. It is a useful thing for a big brunch-type occasion where you have many to feed; make it the day before and pop in the fridge overnight.

To make the yellow omelette, whisk the eggs with the cream and season. Heat a splash of olive oil in a small to medium-sized non-stick pan, add the onion, and to it the soaked saffron. Stir and cook until the onion is translucent. Pour in the whisked eggs and cook until set. When it is totally set, take the omelette off the heat and plate.

To make the green omelette, whisk the eggs and season. Heat the oil in the pan and add the spinach, tarragon and parsley. Add the eggs and the Parmesan and cook until set. Place on top of the yellow omelette.

To make the red omelette, whisk the eggs and season. Heat a splash of olive oil in the pan. Fry the tomatoes for a minute or so, then add the eggs, moving them around with a spatula. Add the goat's cheese and cook until set. Remove and place on top of the green omelette.

Wrap the three omelettes in greaseproof/wax paper and then wrap in a layer of tin foil, pressing them down. Refrigerate overnight and unwrap just before serving with a few more chopped herbs thrown on the top. Cut as you would a cake and serve with a green salad.

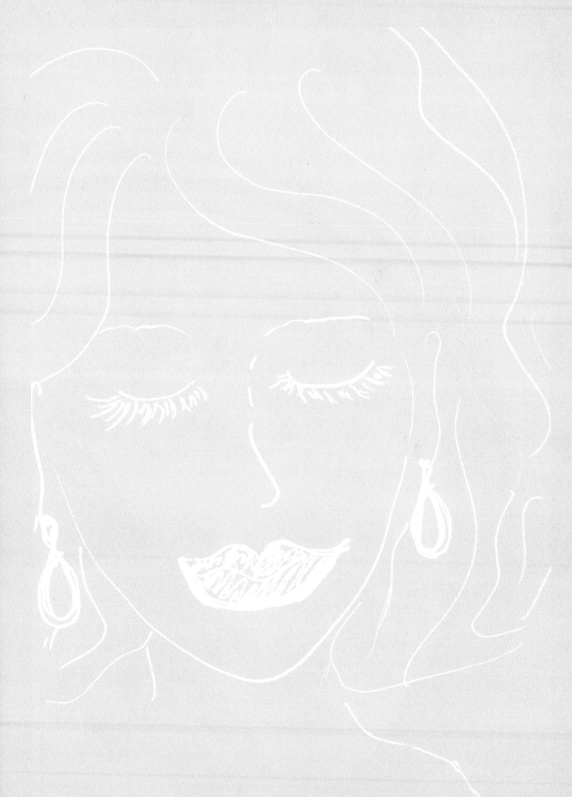

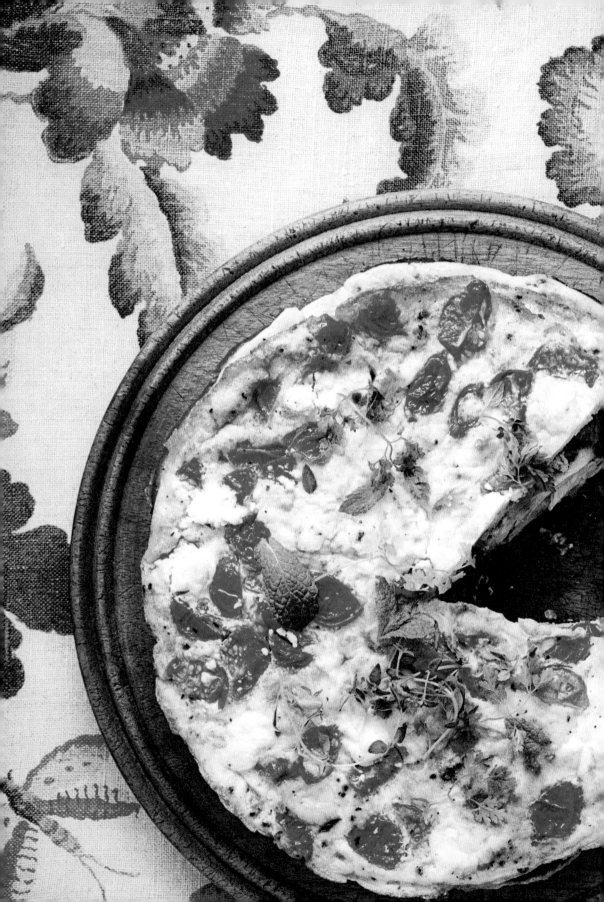

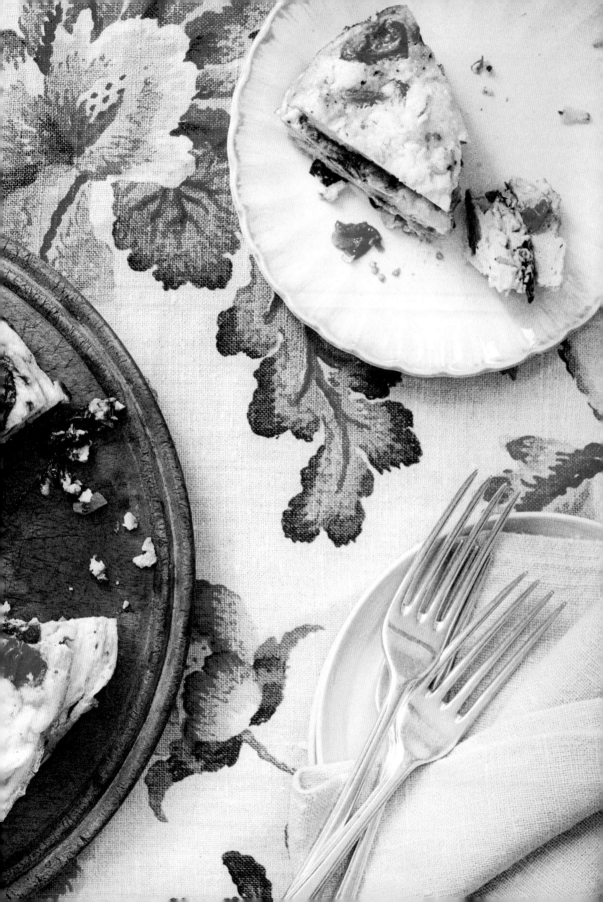

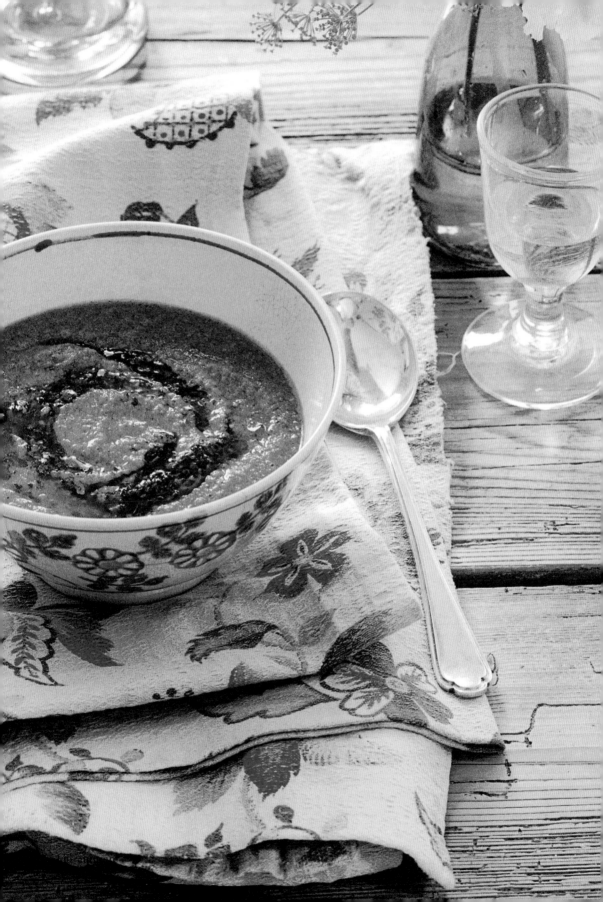

Pea, pesto and rocket/arugula soup

This is quite a useful thing to have in the back of your head if people happen to show up uninvited, although I only ever seem to have eggs in the house when that happens to me, and I have to pretend that, yes, I really did mean to make a frittata for dinner. The soup is dead quick, yet delicious, and hopefully the uninvited will provide their own pudding, or at least have brought some chocolate.

Place all of the pesto ingredients in a blender and whiz up until you have a green, bubbly sauce, adding a splash of water if the pesto is a little thick. Taste, season and adjust anything that needs adjusting.

In a large saucepan, heat the olive oil and soften the onion. Add the courgettes/zucchini, then pour in the stock and simmer on low for 8 to 10 minutes. Add the peas and rocket/arugula, bring back to the boil and cook for another 3 or 4 minutes until tender.

Let the soup cool for 15 minutes or so and then, in careful batches, mix in a blender until you have a velvety purée. Reheat in a saucepan or serve cold, as it works either way. You can either run 4 tablespoons of pesto through the soup when you're serving or reheating, if you are, or if serving cold, add it to the blender when you are puréeing the batches.

SERVES 4

1 tablespoon of olive oil

1 small onion, peeled and finely chopped

2 small courgettes/zucchini, chopped

875ml/3½ cups of chicken or vegetable stock

1 small packet (450g/1lb) of frozen peas

1 large handful of rocket/arugula

For the pesto

1 large handful of fresh basil leaves

1 clove of garlic, peeled and roughly chopped

A few tablespoons of pine nuts

4 tablespoons of olive oil

25g/¼ cup of grated Parmesan

Salt and pepper

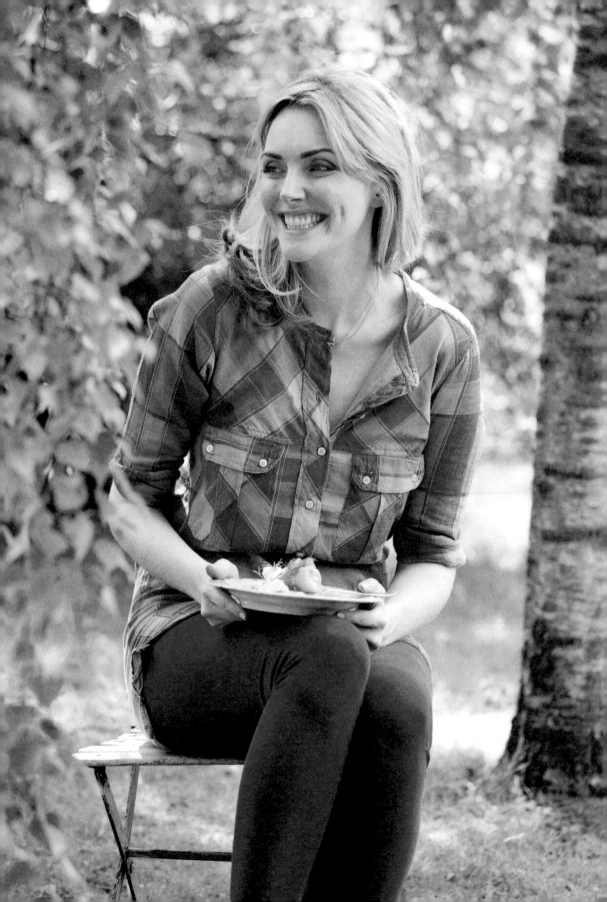

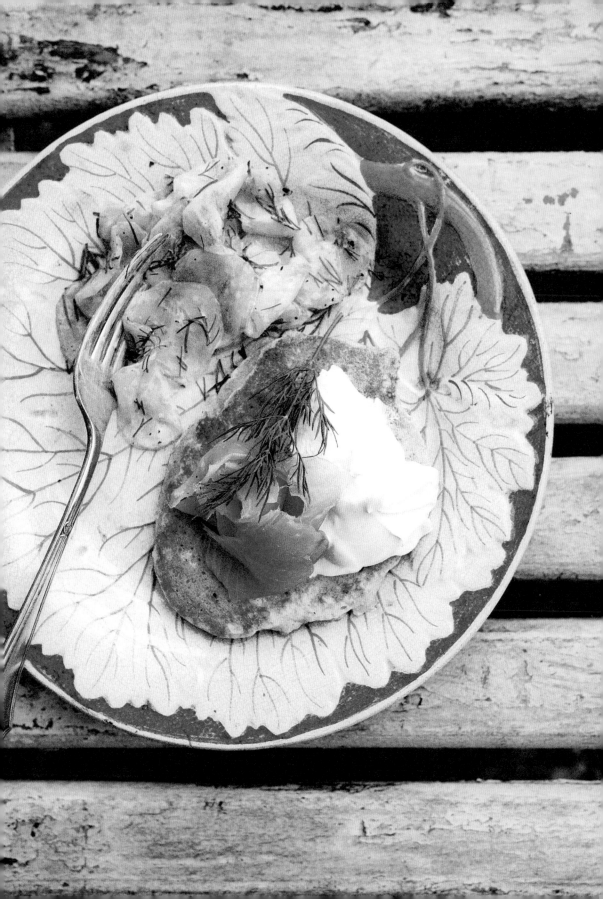

Potato pancakes with smoked salmon and a cucumber and dill salad

MAKES 8 PANCAKES

For the cucumber salad
½ cucumber, peeled and thinly sliced in rounds
1 tablespoon of buttermilk
1 tablespoon of light olive oil
1 teaspoon of white wine vinegar
A squeeze of lemon
Salt and pepper
A small handful of fresh chopped dill

These remind me of being a child. I grew up with a Scottish nanny called Maureen who is not only the best person in the world, but one of the cleverest – boasting a Mensa membership. My brothers and sister and I used to go to Maureen's mum and dad's house in Edinburgh every Hogmanay, until we were too teenage and complaining, and her dad Pop used to make us potato pancakes for breakfast with fried eggs and mushrooms. He also played the bones, and would clack out a tune on the sideboard as the eggs sizzled. We used to steal liqueur chocolates from the sideboard and pretend we were drunk.

Every piece of random general knowledge I possess is from Maureen, and she taught me to tie my shoelaces.

Make the cucumber salad by assembling the cucumber rounds onto a big plate and mixing the buttermilk, olive oil, white wine vinegar, lemon and salt and pepper together into a dressing. Pour over the cucumber and garnish with dill, reserving a bit for the salmon. In a mixing bowl, mix together the mashed potato, flour, bicarb of soda/baking soda and the salt, then beat in the buttermilk. Grate the potato, squeezing out any liquid; add into the mix with the parsley and season.

Heat a griddle pan and melt a knob of butter. Ladle in the potato pancake batter, making individual hotcake-sized rounds. Fry them for about 3 to 5 minutes until burnished and brown, then turn and cook for a couple of minutes longer. Lay the pancakes on a plate, make a curl of salmon on top of each one, dot with crème fraîche and dill and serve the cucumber salad on the side.

For the potato pancakes
125g/⅔ cup of mashed potato
50g/scant ½ cup of spelt flour
¼ teaspoon of bicarbonate of soda/baking soda
Salt and pepper
100ml/scant ½ cup of buttermilk
1 potato (about 100g/3½oz), peeled
A small handful of fresh chopped parsley
A knob of butter

200g/7oz smoked salmon
3 tablespoons of crème fraîche

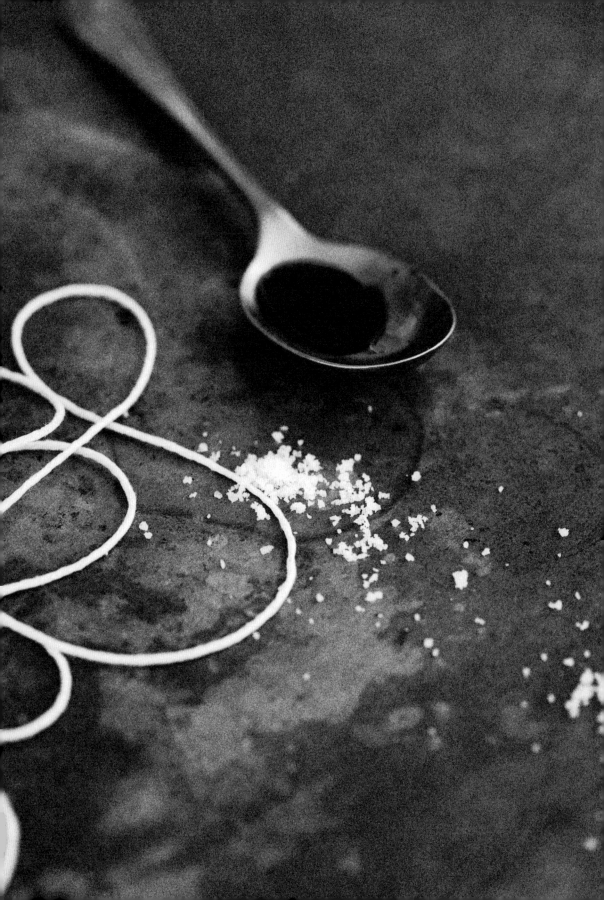

Spring
Suppers

Macky Boy's mackerel
with baby spinach and horseradish dressing

SERVES 2

2 smoked mackerel fillets
1 tablespoon of runny
   honey
A glug of olive oil
2 teaspoons of capers

For the salad
1 tablespoon of olive oil
1 teaspoon of white wine
   vinegar
1 heaped teaspoon of
   fresh finely grated
   horseradish
A squeeze of lemon
2 heaped tablespoons of
   crème fraîche
Salt and pepper
2 handfuls of baby spinach

My friend and neighbour Mac is a photographer by trade, but he also cooks a mean dinner, and the ladies love him for it. If I'm feeling particularly deluded, I start feeling a bit Wendy to the Lost Boys and will cook for the entire street. Sometimes this extends to cooking Mac a fry up, as he gets a very hungry, haunted look in the morning. He cooked me mackerel brushed with honey to return the favour, and it turned into this. He tells me that my crumble is 'Article lick!' and like a lot of West Indian and island sayings, it sings what it means. I think this is one of the best compliments I have ever received. This saying has been shortened in my house to 'It's the lick', when something's brilliant.

Preheat the oven to 200°C/180°C fan/Gas 6. Place the mackerel on some foil on an oven tray. Brush the mackerel on either side with the honey and place in the hot oven. Cook for 10 minutes or so.

In the meantime, heat a glug of the olive oil in a small frying pan and when it's searing hot, add the capers. Fry the capers until they are crispy. For the salad, make the dressing by mixing together the oil and vinegar and slowly whisking in the horseradish, lemon and crème fraîche. Season to taste, then dress the spinach. Alternatively, serve the horseradish on the side as a cream by slowly whisking the horseradish and lemon into the crème fraîche instead of the dressing and seasoning to taste. Serve the crispy mackerel on top of the spinach, dotted with the capers and accompanied by the horseradish cream if making.

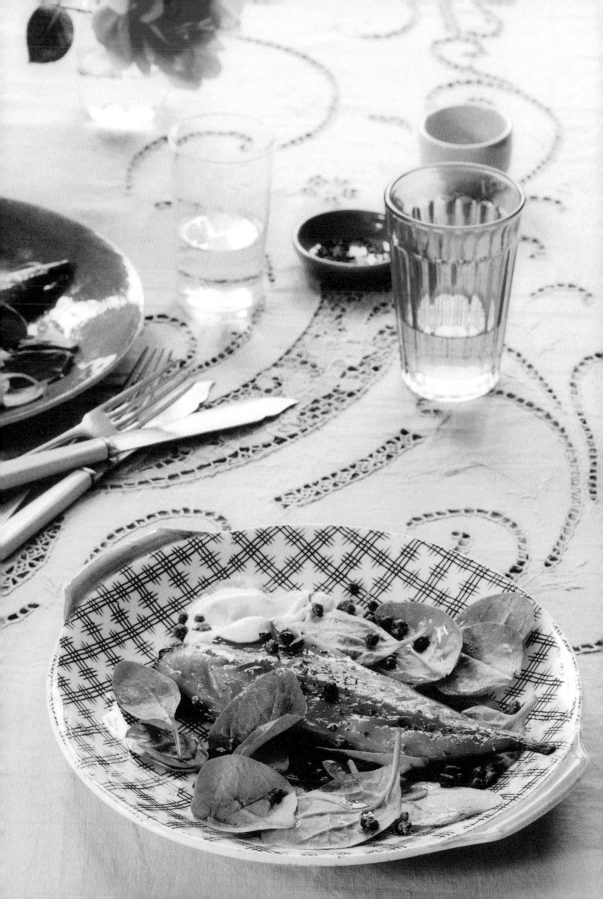

Coconut and crab rice with lime and coriander/cilantro

SERVES 2

1 tablespoon of sunflower
  oil
1 teaspoon of coriander
  seeds
1 teaspoon of cumin seeds
  or ground cumin
1 small onion, peeled and
  finely chopped
1 small red chilli, deseeded
  and finely chopped
1 spring onion/scallion,
  finely chopped
250ml/1 cup of coconut
  milk
250ml/1 cup of fish stock
275g/1½ cups of basmati
  rice
Salt and pepper
170g/¾ cup of cooked
  white crab meat
1 small handful of fresh
  coriander/cilantro,
  chopped
Juice and zest of 1 lime

This is another one of those easy spring dishes. You could also run a tablespoon of yoghurt through for some cool amongst the chilli.

In a medium-sized saucepan (with a tight-fitting lid), heat the oil. Add to it the coriander seeds and the cumin, then the onion, chilli and spring onion/scallion. Stir for a few minutes, coating with the spicy oil. Pour in the coconut milk and fish stock and add the rice. Season, bring to a rolling boil and, as soon as this has happened, put the lid on and bring the heat right down. Cook for 10 minutes. Take off the heat, fluff and add the crab meat, chopped coriander and juice and zest of the lime. Serve.

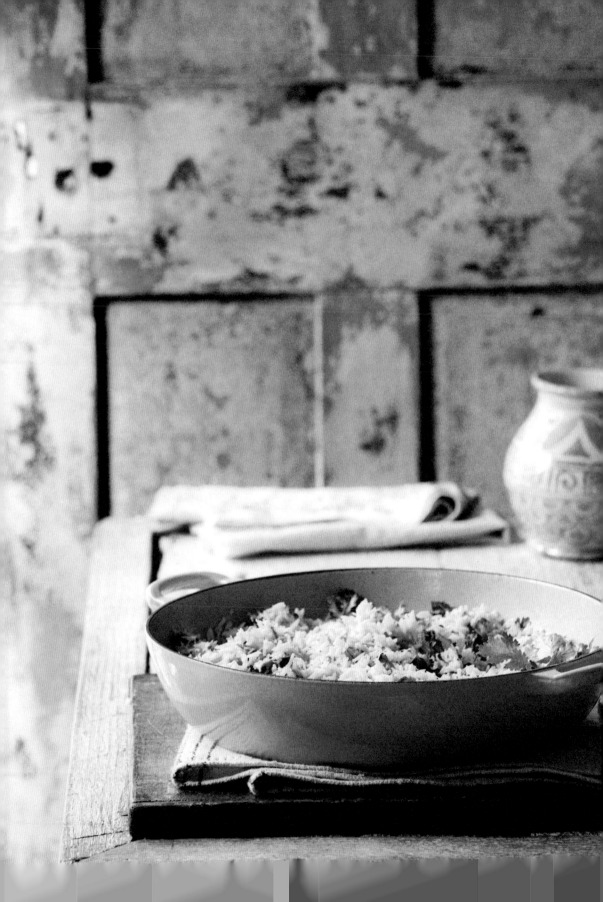

Pollack with Indian spices and yoghurt lime dressing

A fragrant way to tart up a piece of fish. Serve with basmati rice tempered with a cardamom pod or two, and some steamed, buttered spinach. If you finish with rose petal ice cream, you're in for a happy night.

Put the whole spices in a small frying pan and dry-roast over a medium heat for a couple of minutes until they smell aromatic. Transfer them to a pestle and mortar, add the ginger, cinnamon, salt and pepper and bash together until you have a rough powder. Rub this mix into the pollack and leave to one side.

Make the yoghurt dressing by mixing the yoghurt, lime juice and zest and coriander/cilantro together in a small mixing bowl. Season to taste.

Heat a griddle pan until searing and place the pollack on it, cooking for about 4 minutes on each side. Serve with rice and a salad, with the yoghurt dressing draping off the pollack.

SERVES 4

1 teaspoon of coriander
　seeds
1 teaspoon of cumin seeds
1 teaspoon of fenugreek
　seeds
½ teaspoon of ground
　ginger
A pinch of ground
　cinnamon
Sea salt and a few black
　peppercorns
4 pollack fillets

For the yoghurt dressing
4–6 tablespoons of Greek
　yoghurt, strained
Juice and grated zest of
　1 lime
1 small handful of fresh
　finely chopped
　coriander/cilantro
Salt and pepper

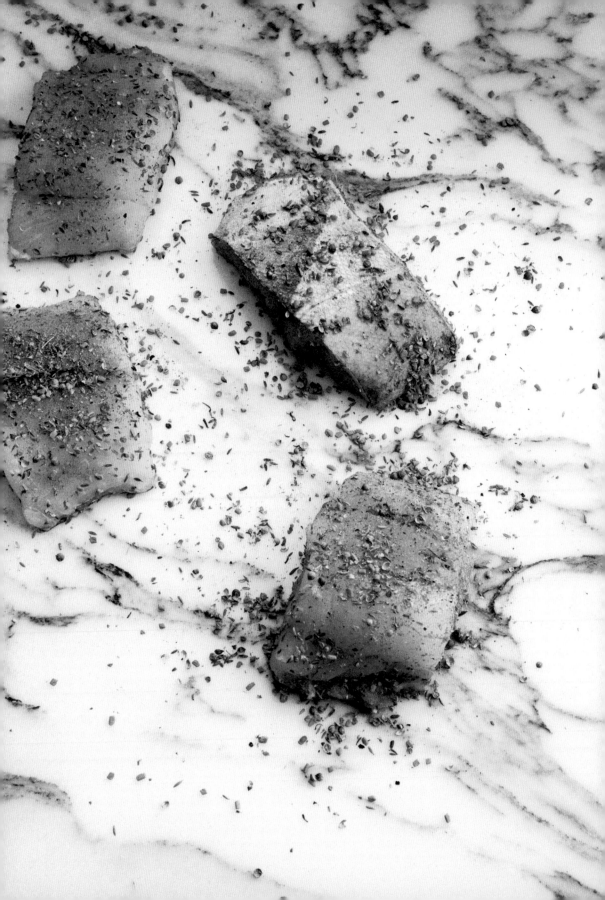

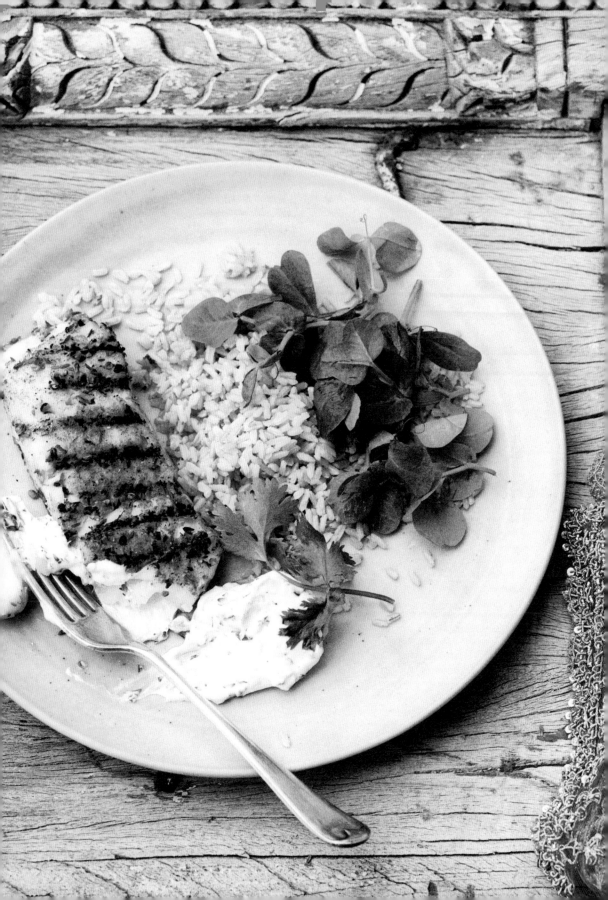

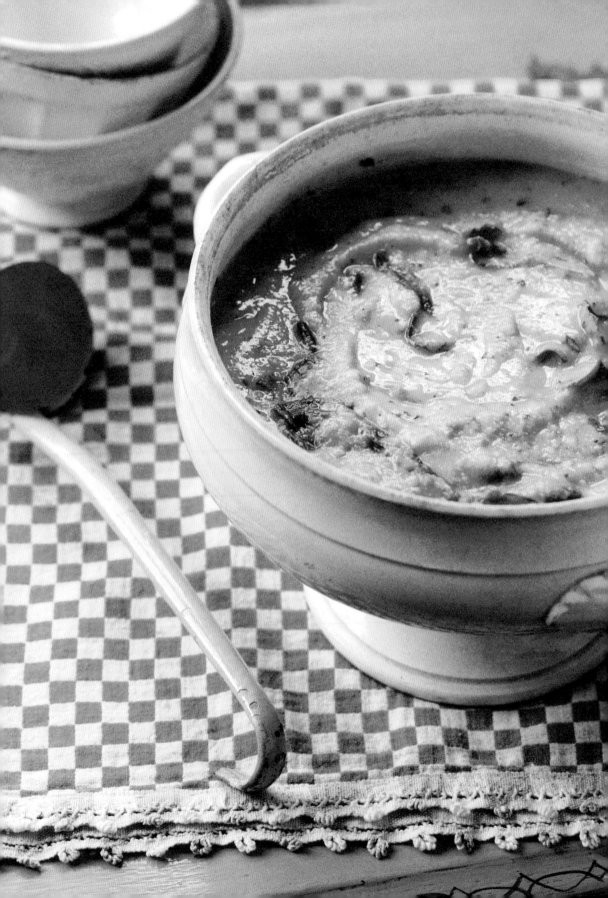

Lemon lentil soup

I was inspired to make this after going to a Persian restaurant late at night and eating a lentil soup heavy with lemon. Theirs was hot, and quite thin. I liked the idea of making it almost like a stew, something you could possibly toss some rice and yoghurt into, with lots of coriander. It's a meal in itself and I also like that kind of one-stop eating.

In a large, heavy-bottomed pot, cover the lentils with 1 litre of stock and add the bay leaves. Bring to the boil, and then simmer on low, uncovered, for 30 to 40 minutes until very soft.

While the lentils are cooking, heat the olive oil in a frying pan. Gently sweat the onion and spring onions/scallions on low for around 10 minutes, and then add the celery. Sprinkle the cumin on and stir, heating for another 5 minutes or so and adding a little more olive oil if necessary. Add this mix to the lentils with the lemon juice. Remove the bay leaves and season to taste.

Let everything cool for a bit, then transfer to a blender, adding the extra stock or water to get it soupy. Depending on the size of your blender, you may have to do this in two batches.

Pour the soup back into the washed saucepan and reheat on low, adding the spinach and half the coriander/cilantro. Season to taste again.

Serve at room temperature with some more lemon juice and olive oil, the remaining coriander/cilantro and, if you have some, a swirl of Greek yoghurt.

SERVES 6

500g/2 cups of red lentils

1 litre/4 cups of vegetable or chicken stock, plus 250ml/1 cup of stock or water

3 bay leaves

2 tablespoons of olive oil, plus extra for serving

½ onion, peeled and finely chopped

2 spring onions/scallions, white part only, finely chopped

2 celery sticks, finely chopped

1 tablespoon of ground cumin

Juice of 3 lemons, plus extra for serving

Salt and pepper

100g/2 cups of spinach, roughly chopped

20g/¾oz fresh coriander/cilantro, finely chopped

Paella

4 tablespoons of olive oil

4 skinless and boneless
  chicken breasts, cut into
  bite-sized pieces

100g/3½oz of chorizo,
  sliced

1 onion, peeled and finely
  chopped

3 cloves of garlic, peeled
  and finely chopped

A large pinch of saffron

1.2 litres/5 cups of chicken
  stock

500g/2 cups of Spanish
  short-grain paella rice

¼ teaspoon of dried red
  chilli flakes

4 large tomatoes,
  deseeded and chopped

8 or so king prawns/jumbo
  shrimp

8 or so scallops

310g/2 cups of frozen peas

A handful of fresh parsley

1 lemon, cut into wedges

Good paella can be a bit of a Holy Grail, and everyone argues about what should go into it. Given that I don't eat chorizo, I should probably not add my voice to the clamour, for the risk of being stoned. But here it is anyway, inspired by a trip to Barcelona and an old-fashioned seafood restaurant with green tiles and smoky mirrors.

Heat a tablespoon of the oil in a big deep frying pan and pan-fry the chicken breast until browned, adding the chorizo to cook for the last few minutes. Add the onion and the garlic and sweat for another few minutes. Mix the saffron into your warm stock and let it infuse for a couple of minutes. Adding more oil to the pan, stir in the rice and pour in half of the saffron-infused stock. Add the chilli and tomatoes and cook on a lowish heat for around 20 minutes, stirring occasionally.

Just towards the end, add the rest of the chicken stock and the prawns/shrimp and scallops and cook for another 5 minutes with a lid on the pan. Lastly, add the peas and cook for another 4 minutes or so. Serve with heaped parsley, a dash of olive oil and a wedge of lemon.

Chicken Kiev

I was talking with some friends about nostalgic food from childhood. Sherbet dips, Hula-Hoops and that ubiquitous menu staple from the 80s, the Chicken Kiev. We all agreed that the advent of Chicken Kiev was about the most exciting thing ever; that first slice into the plump chicken breast, followed by a hot waft of garlic and pool of molten green butter. I wondered whether you could make a healthy one, and was there even a point? Having trialled this, I think so, and friends' kids might even agree…

Preheat the oven to 200°C/180°C fan/Gas 6.

Make a mixture of the houmous, olive oil and parsley and leave to the side. Don't over mix as you don't want the oil too incorporated into the houmous. With a very sharp knife, make a narrow slice through the side of the chicken breasts. This will create a small pocket in which to stuff the houmousy mixture. Push this in with a spoon and then close with your fingers. Put the stuffed chicken breasts in the fridge and leave for half an hour.

When you take them out, dredge each breast with spelt flour, brush with the beaten egg and then coat with the rye breadcrumbs. Take a large frying pan, heat a glug of olive oil and fry the breasts for a few minutes until they are evenly golden. Transfer to a baking tray and bake for 20 minutes.

SERVES 4

4 tablespoons of houmous
2 tablespoons of olive oil
A small handful of fresh chopped parsley
4 skinless, boneless chicken breasts
3 tablespoons of spelt flour
1 egg, beaten
100g/1 cup of rye breadcrumbs

The Sheriff's marinated lamb

SERVES 6

Leg of lamb (about
   2kg/4½lb)
A small handful of fresh
   finely chopped rosemary
1 teaspoon of mustard
   powder
Finely chopped fresh
   ginger (about
   2 tablespoons worth)
1 teaspoon of soy sauce
1 small handful of fresh
   chopped mint
1 teaspoon of white wine
   vinegar
1 teaspoon of
   demerara/raw
   brown sugar
3 cloves of garlic, peeled

Everyone kept telling me that my father-in-law, John, had an incredible lamb recipe. I rang him, my culinary detective nose on the hunt.

'May I have your incredible lamb recipe for my book?' I asked.

'Lamb recipe? Do I have one?' He answered, shades of Mor Mor sending my heart to my boots. It turned out, after much haranguing, that he actually did, but it was mostly in his head. Whilst he will not win awards for his recipe writing, which I have adapted here (big difference between an hour to two and a bit), he may win one for the lamb itself, being an all-round good egg and the High Sheriff of Bath, thank you very much, and finally, along with his friend Dave, for being the most devoted Swindon Town supporter ever.

Put the leg in a large roasting tray. The lamb is best marinated for at least 2 hours, so make the marinade before you do anything else. Place the rosemary in a large pestle and mortar with all the other ingredients, except the garlic. Give it a good grind and then, with your fingers, massage the marinade into the lamb. Chop your garlic cloves into little spears and push them into the meat where you want them. Leave the lamb covered, somewhere cool, for 2 hours; more, if you have time. About half an hour before cooking, preheat the oven to 230°C/210°C fan/Gas 8. When the oven is hot enough, put the lamb in and roast for 20 minutes, after which you're going to turn the oven down to 200°C/180°C fan/Gas 6. Cook for about another hour and 20 minutes for lamb that is juicy and pink in the middle. Another 15 minutes more if you like it well done. Once you have removed from the oven, let the lamb rest for about 10 minutes before carving.

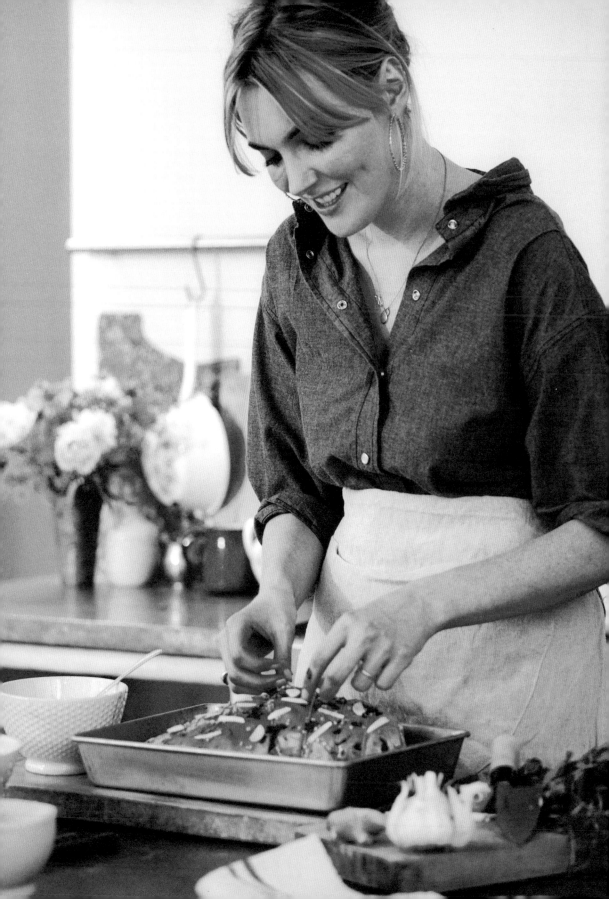

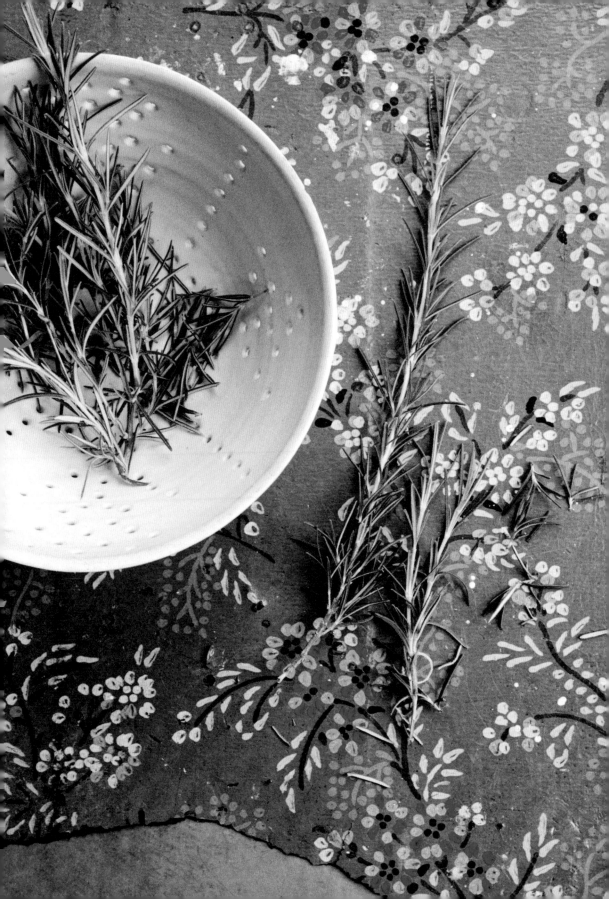

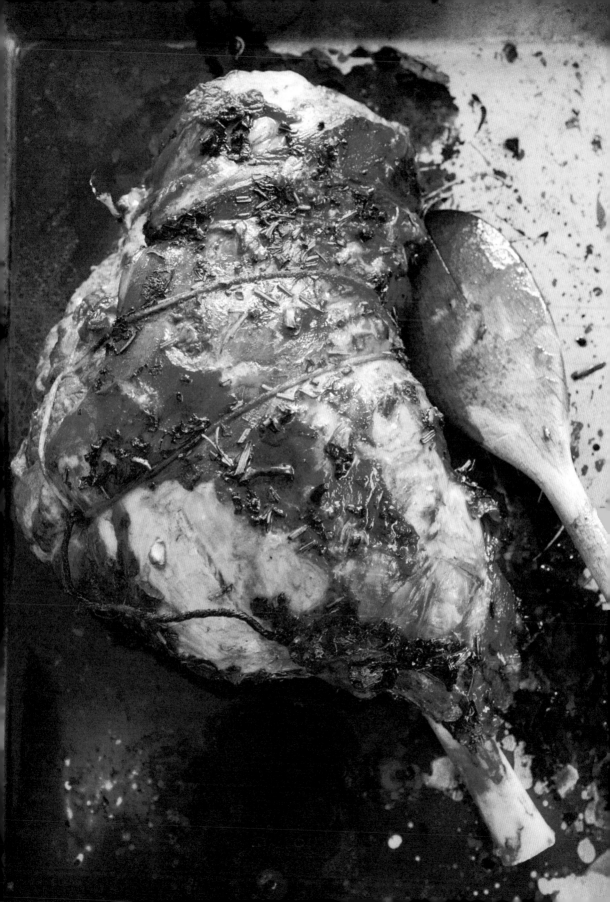

Come sit with me in the shade.......

Summer

BREAKFASTS
Fruit salad with orange flower syrup and mint
Grilled peaches with ricotta and toasted pistachios
Tomato tofu basil scramble
Rory's savoury pancakes that are not a breakfast cake
Fennel frittata
Strawberry pancakes
Carrot and cream cheese muffins

LUNCHES
Sheep's cheese with flaming ouzo
Tzatziki
Radishes with truffle salt and mint and olive oil
Ceviche with prawns/shrimp and avocado
Grilled octopus with potatoes and fagiolini bean pesto
Kebabs
Raw golden beetroot/beets with cayenne and lime

SUPPERS
Ricotta tarts with creamy pecorino sauce and shavings of black
   truffle
Chicken summer stew
Roasted tomato mascarpone soup with basil oil
Courgette/zucchhini flower risotto
Miso black Colin
Rowley Leigh's Parmesan custard with anchovy toast and a herb
   salad (all mine)
Broad bean/fava risotto

There is something lulling and rhythmic about August. The summer has sloped into its routine and everyone has, by then, either found their feet or lost their shoes. It is a time for brief, heady love. If you're a teenager, perhaps with a person whose language escapes you, but whose eyes say it all. If you are older, but maybe not wiser, it's a place, a meal, a time, which swoops you up and makes you giddy, cradling you in the transient cup of infatuation. It was famously written about, this summer malady, in books from *Tender is the Night* to *Bonjour Tristesse*, and captured in a jam jar with Joss, the heroine of *The Greengage Summer*. Everything seems possible in the summer: love, escape and even loss. Grief feels wrong in the heat.

In hot lapses, I've fallen in love with houses that I will never see again, stolen a wooden sailboat (and returned it), and briefly written my life into a town that is now a murmur of Italian that I can't quite hear. All in the name of summer. It is cathartic; this once-a-year release, where you can shed your skin under an olive grove, or on a pier with a big wheel blaring colour and pop songs.

The food of summer is equally memorable; ambling lunches eaten outside, a table with grilled meats and vegetables with smoky sauces, followed by plates of plump strawberries and peaches and light-as-air lemon mousse. Or the sharp sting of vinegar on fish and chips, demolished on a stone wall by a shingle beach, cold beer the perfect mate to it. Vanilla ice cream was made to be guzzled after swimming in the sea, the salt on your fingers tempering the sugar. It's hard to pick a favourite summer food memory, but up there would be the lobster and crabs legs we ate on my brother's birthday, on a tiny wooden deck in a fishing port in Massachusetts. We ate from paper plates, with tubs of melted butter and a great mess of coleslaw and summer corn on the side. His girlfriend had made some gooey fudge brownies, and they finished the feast. All my summer food memories seem to contain a brownie at the end; last summer no exception.

I had the total luxury of being on a small fishing boat off the coast of Dorset in England with the wonderful cook Hugh Fearnley-Whittingstall and his fishing partner, Nick Fisher. It was my husband

and I and a small group of friends. It was a rare cloudless day, the sort that Laurie Lee would write of. We fished for mackerel, which are abundant in those waters, and ate them as sashimi, thinly sliced with a smear of wasabi. Some hours later we came across some scallop divers who sold us a few of their trove. Those we cooked on an open grill on the half shell, with some wild garlic, lemon zest and chilli, a hunk of sourdough bread, fresh baked that morning, to sop up the juice.

I don't remember who suggested the swim; I think it began as a dare as the waters that far out, even in July, are pretty arctic. If we were to undertake it, the prize was a brownie, molten and dense with a steaming cup of tea. Hugh dove in like an otter, dipping under the boat for an anxious minute. I was in my knickers and an old t-shirt and I teetered on the edge of the boat. I took a deep breath and surrendered, disappearing into water so cold that I swore like a sailor when I finally came up to meet the surface. The brownie that heralded the shuddering return to the boat was manna, the strong tea its perfect partner.

On the drive home, we splayed out in the car; freckled, salt-stained and replete. Nick Drake sang 'Pink Moon' on the radio. It was how life should be.

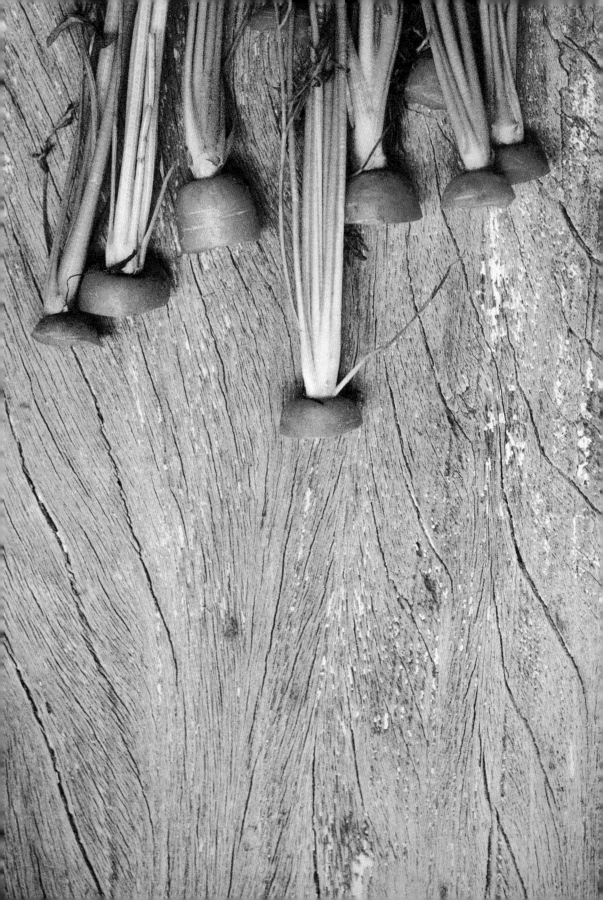

Summer
Breakfasts

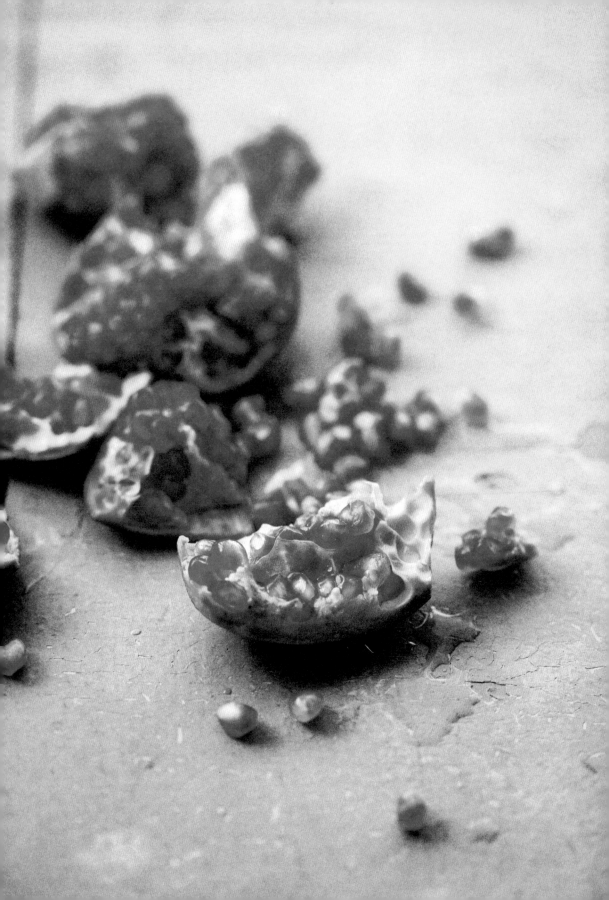

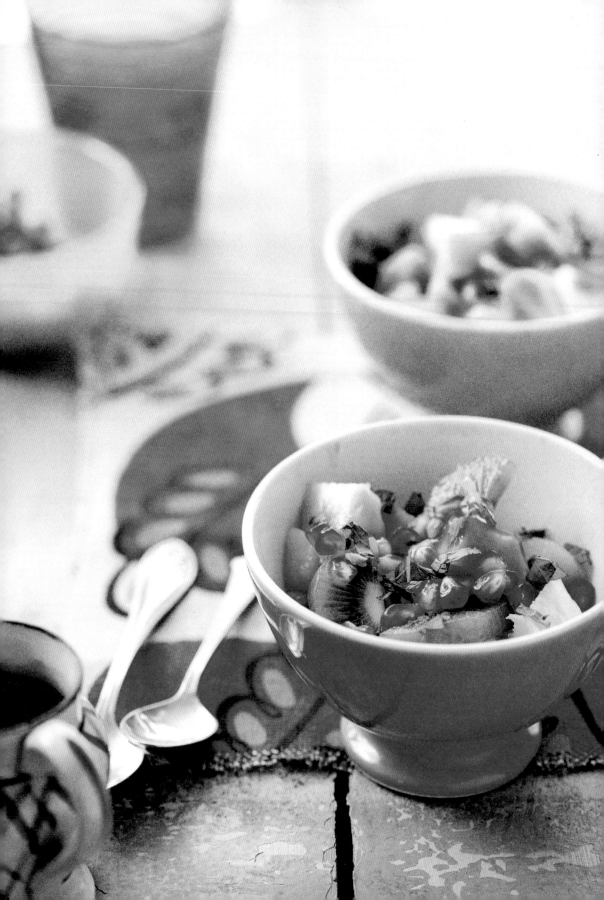

Fruit salad with orange flower syrup and mint

SERVES 2–4

1 kiwi, peeled and chopped

½ a small pineapple, chopped into bite-sized pieces

1 ripe mango, chopped

The seeds of 1 pomegranate

½ a papaya/pawpaw, deseeded and chopped

A handful of fresh mint

For the syrup

2 tablespoons of water

1 tablespoon of agave syrup or honey

1 teaspoon of orange flower water

Does what it says on the box. However, the syrup is also really good poured on a lemon cake that's a day or two old.

First, make the syrup in a small pan on a low to medium heat. Add the water, agave or honey and orange flower water and simmer, reducing for a few minutes until you have a syrup. Leave to the side and cool. Put the chopped fruit in a bowl deserving of it. Chop the mint and add it to the mix, lastly pouring the cooled syrup on top. Voila!

Grilled peaches with ricotta and toasted pistachios

I love grilling or roasting fruit. It brings out a latent cushiony sweetness that is perfectly met with cheese or crème fraîche. Also works wonders when you're looking for a light, summery pudding.

Preheat a griddle pan until very hot or heat the grill. Rub the peaches with a bit of butter. Place them on the pan and sear for a few minutes on either side, until soft and juicy on the inside and golden on the out. Plate and drizzle with runny honey and the ricotta. In the still-hot pan, toast the pistachios for a minute or so and pour over the peaches.

SERVES 2

2 peaches, stoned and
   halved
A knob of butter
1 tablespoon of runny dark
   honey
2 tablespoons of ricotta
   cheese
1 handful of shelled
   unsalted pistachios

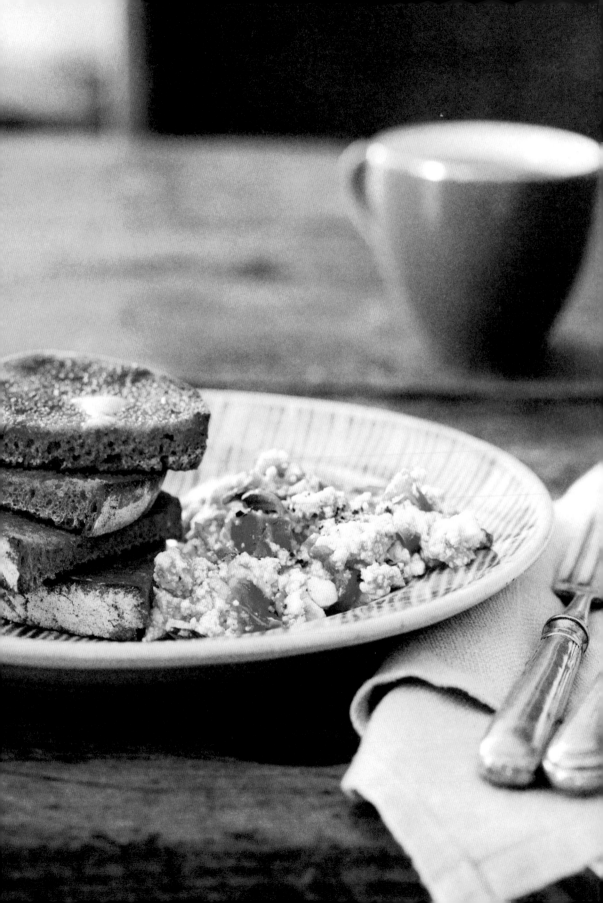

Tomato tofu basil scramble

Some people are appalled by tofu. I don't know this, but I imagine Adrian Gill is; in a laconic, laid-back sort of way. Clarissa Dickson Wright would point blank ignore it, possibly making it sit in the corner, and Gordon Ramsay would set it on fire, calling it a bastard. I am not appalled by tofu. I like it very much, particularly scrambled on toast.

Heat the oil in a pan and add the garlic, stirring for a minute. Add the tomatoes and basil, and cook on low for another 2 minutes. Add the passata. Crumble in the tofu and the feta and mix it all through, adding a little vegetable stock if it starts to look dry. Taste and season accordingly.

SERVES 1

1 tablespoon of olive oil

1 clove of garlic, peeled and finely chopped

4 medium/large heirloom tomatoes, chopped

A handful of fresh roughly torn basil

1 tablespoon of passata

160g/about ½ a block of firm tofu

30g/¼ cup of crumbled feta

A splash of vegetable stock

Salt and pepper

Rory's savoury pancakes that are not a breakfast cake

SERVES 2

For the filling
2 handfuls of spinach
Olive oil
110g/½ a cup of soft goat's
  cheese
A small handful of fresh
  finely chopped parsley,
Salt and pepper

For the pancakes
115g/1 cup of spelt flour
1 egg
125ml/½ cup of milk
2 tablespoons of olive oil

I was on a very noisy bus with Rory, who plays the trumpet. We were travelling through Germany, talking about food.

'Can I have a recipe named after me in your book?' He said.

'Yes. Do you want a savoury breakfast crêpe named after you? I've got one of those going spare.' I said.

He got very excited.

'Yes! Yes! A breakfast cake! What's in it?'

At that moment our bus was stopped and searched by some very polite German policemen, so the conversation ended there. We assured them we were not drug smugglers, they took our word for it, and that was that. The breakfast cake was never mentioned again, until now.

Sorry, this is not a breakfast cake, Roar.

First make the filling. In a frying pan, wilt the spinach with a little bit of olive oil. Cool and then put in a blender with the goat's cheese, parsley and some salt and pepper to taste and whiz until blended.

Make the pancake batter by mixing the flour, egg, milk and a tablespoon of olive oil together until you have a smooth batter. Heat another tablespoon of olive oil in a frying pan and add a ladleful of batter. You want the pancakes to be thick enough to hold the filling but not so fat that they are lumpy – a sort of plumped-up crêpe. When they are brown and lacy on each side, remove them from the heat, add the filling and roll them up.

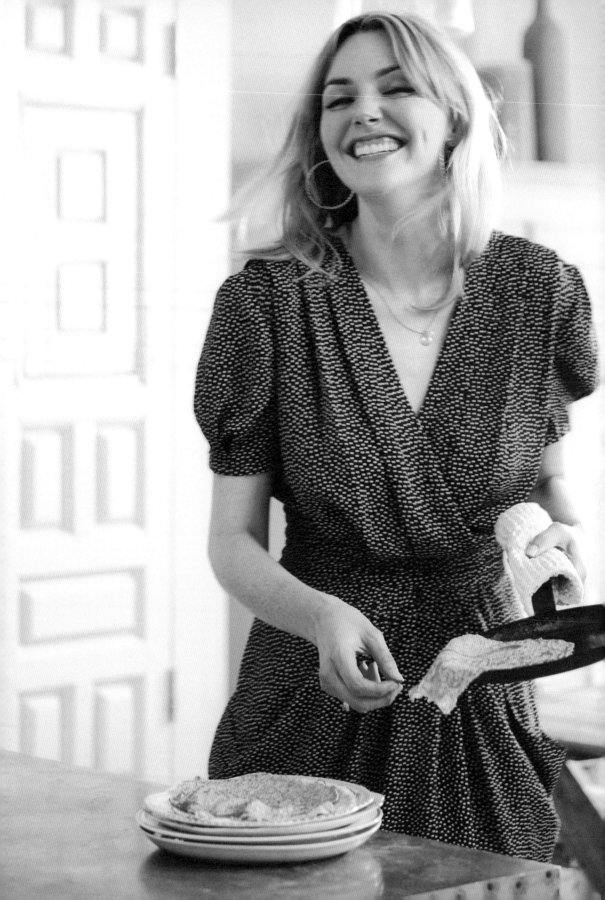

Fennel frittata

SERVES 2

4 eggs
1 fennel bulb, with a few of
   the fronds
2 tablespoons of olive oil
Salt and pepper 20g/¼ cup
   or so of grated Parmesan

Fennel is a generous, diplomatic vegetable that works pretty much anywhere. Conjure up *The Talented Mr Ripley*, pre all the murderous action, and eat this pretending you're on the Amalfi Coast. You can serve it cold and with a tomato salad for lunch or supper too.

Preheat the grill to High and whisk the eggs.

Peel the tough outer leaves of the fennel and discard. Shave the inside so you have thin ribbons, and then further chop it down so it is in bite-sized pieces.

Heat a frying pan and add the olive oil, and then add the fennel. Stir for a few minutes, until the colour turns slightly and then add the whisked eggs and salt and pepper. Cook until the bottom sets, sprinkle with the grated Parmesan and then pop under the grill until risen and triumphant, which should take about 3 or 4 minutes at most. Serve quickly, garnished with a few fennel fronds.

Strawberry pancakes

The first cook book I ever owned was *The Winnie the Pooh Cook Book*, and in it was a lovely recipe for pancakes. They are universally appealing and there remains something childishly pleasing about finding fruit in them. I like blueberries here too.

In a mixing bowl, mix together the ricotta, milk and egg yolks. Sieve in the flour and baking powder.

In a separate bowl, whisk the egg whites and, just before they are stiff, fold them into the first mixing bowl.

Heat the oil in a frying pan until hot and drop in the batter in 8–10cm/3–4 inch circles. When it begins to look pinpricked, sprinkle some strawberries into the pancake and, when set, turn it. They should take about 2 minutes on each side. Serve with more strawberries and some maple syrup.

SERVES 2

225g/1 cup of ricotta cheese
125ml/½ cup of milk
2 eggs, separated
115g/1 cup of spelt flour
1 teaspoon of baking powder
2 tablespoons of vegetable oil
A handful of strawberries, finely chopped
Maple syrup, to serve

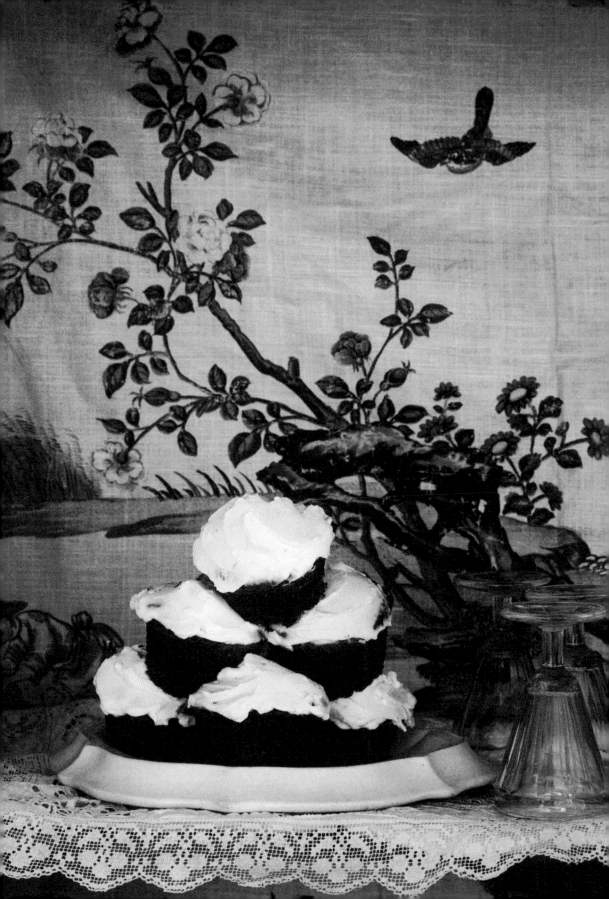

Carrot and cream cheese muffins

I suppose that this is a bit of an excuse to have what is really a cake, in pretend, pseudo-healthy breakfast form. Sometimes life calls for breakfast cake, it just does, especially when you are pregnant and your legs hurt and your feet have grown a whole size.

Preheat the oven to 190°C/170°C fan/Gas 5.

Cream the eggs, sugar and sunflower oil with an electric whisk until incorporated. In a separate bowl, sieve the self-raising flour, bicarbonate of soda/baking soda and spices together. Roughly chop the walnuts and add to the dry ingredients along with the grated carrots. Fold the dry ingredients into the creamed egg mixture and slowly combine with the warm water.

Spoon the mixture into one or two oiled muffin trays and bake for 25 minutes. For the cream cheese icing, whisk together the cream cheese, icing/confectioners' sugar and vanilla essence, then add the lemon juice and zest.

When the muffins are cool, ice with the cream cheese icing and sprinkle with cinnamon.

MAKES 12

2 eggs

200g/scant 1 cup of caster/superfine sugar

185ml/¾ cup of sunflower oil

160g/1¼ cups of self-raising (self-rising) flour

1 teaspoon of bicarbonate of soda/baking soda

2 teaspoons of cinnamon

2 teaspoons of mixed spice

50g/½ cup of walnuts

235g/1½ cups of grated carrots

80ml/⅓ cup of warm water

Ground cinnamon, to dust

For the cream cheese icing

250g/1 cup of cream cheese

60g/¼ cup of icing sugar/confectioners' sugar

Vanilla essence/extract

Zest and juice of 1 lemon

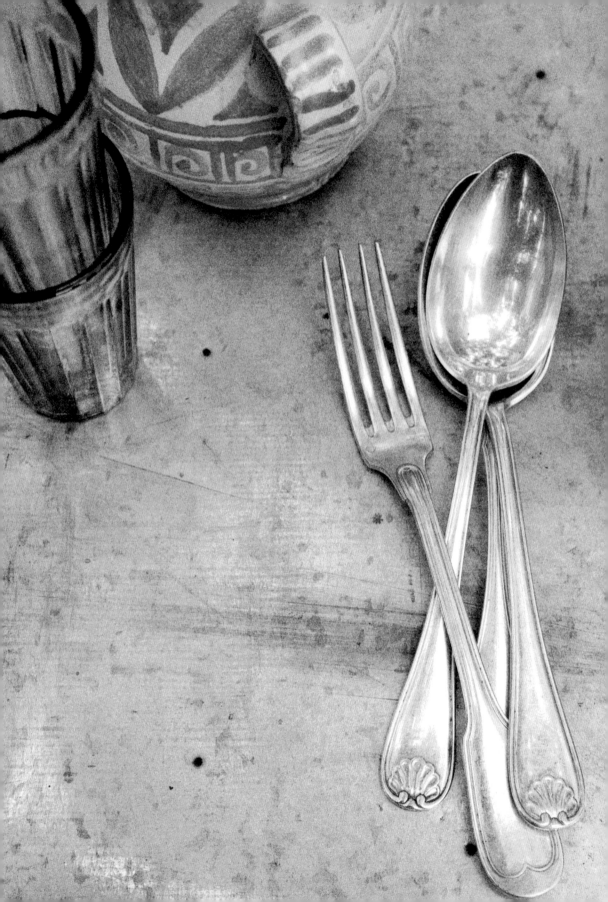

Summer
Lunches

Big fat feast

There are few things better than a great heaving table in the garden of a summer, particularly when it's a table filled with things you actually want to eat. I'm sure British readers will remember with a wry smile the lukewarm picnic offerings of years gone by, an indelibly comic part of some English summers: quease-inducing coronation chicken; the ubiquitous poached salmon, spiked with flecks of cucumber and an army of bones to choke the vicar; eggs of dubious age suspended in melting aspic; warm Pimms; and Eton Mess left out to curdle and splay, a bit like the skirt of a gin-breathed teacher riding dangerously high from the egg and spoon race.

But a summer table filled with delicious choice and Mediterranean influences; now that's a table I can get with. One of the dishes in this section, the octopus, green bean and potato salad, comes straight from the epicentre of this type of eating, its provenance the kitchen of a magical small hotel in Umbria. Others are transported from happy memory to the page: tzatziki made by a big mama in an enormous swimming costume on a small fishing boat off the coast of Greece; radishes from the farmer's market cut wafer thin and dusted with truffle salt and mint (don't panic, truffle salt is relatively inexpensive, and is a fiscally manageable way to conjure up the real thing); kebabs held in sticky fingers, dripping with a garlicky almond dressing; golden beetroot hot with cayenne; ceviche, conjuring Mexico (for an island flavour, add a dash of coconut milk); and salted sheep's cheese flamed with the aniseed magic of Ouzo. I'm convinced the flaming sheep's cheese we ate in a restaurant in Los Angeles is what sent my sister Clover into labour, and immediately after having her son, my gorgeous nephew Finley, she called to find out where we could get some more, and how quickly.

What to drink with this medley? God, anything from a beer with a wedge of lime to a sparkling pinot noir. For the teetotaller, a pink lemonade or iced tea made with Earl Grey or Jasmine tea would do very well. You don't need a garden or a big table to serve it on – a rug on the floor would do just as well, and you'll be safe from wasps and that bit closer to the large nap that you'll need anyway.

For me, each of these things contains the very essence of summer, whether you're home or away.

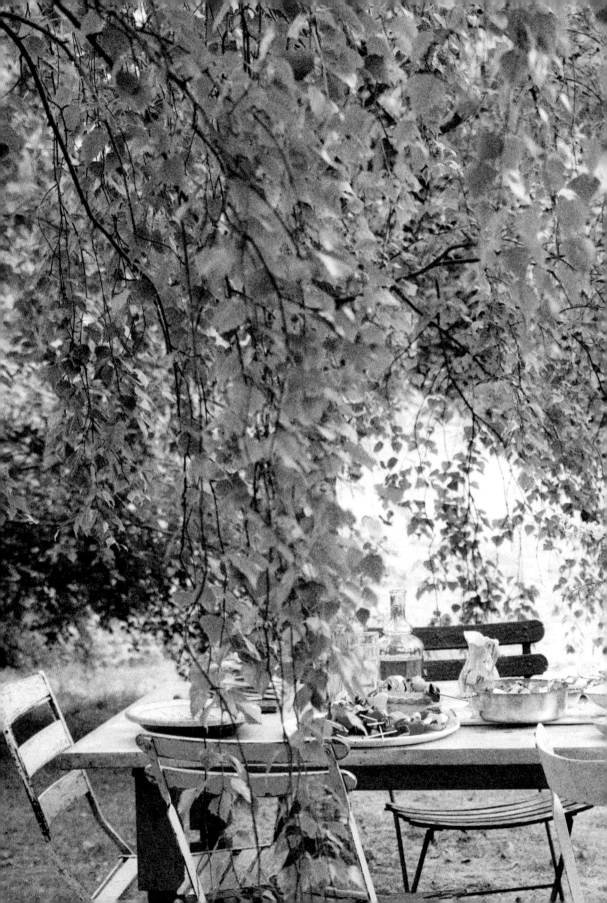

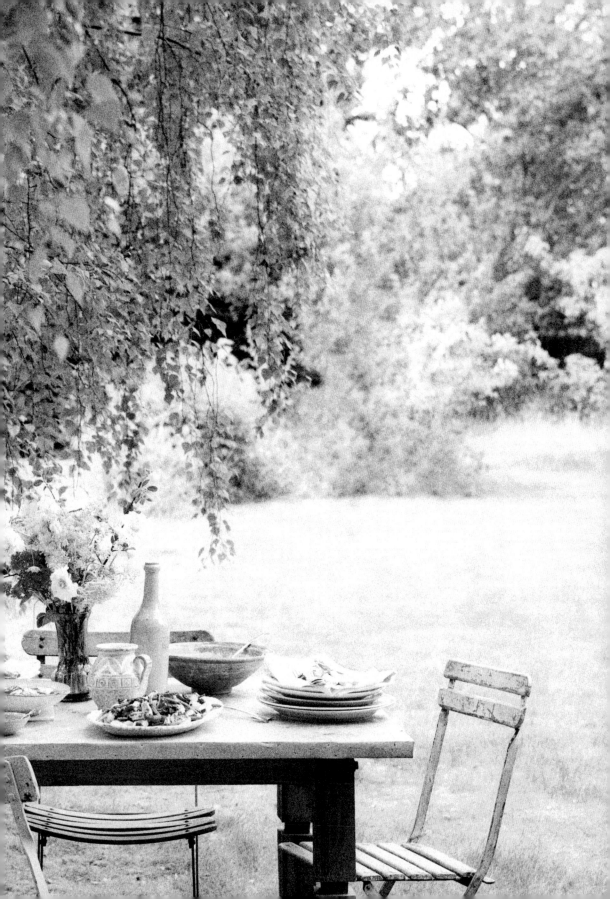

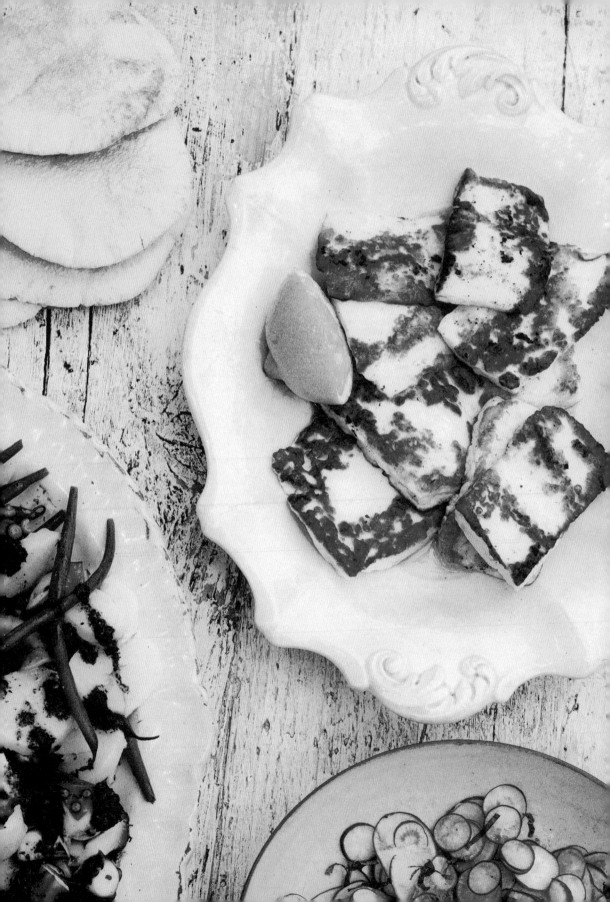

Sheep's cheese with flaming ouzo

You want to use a hard sheep's cheese here, something like Greek Kasseri.

I would recommend doing this in a big non-stick frying pan. Heat the pan until searing, brush with a few drops of olive oil and put the cheese in. Sizzle! Cook it on both sides until golden brown and crispy at the edges. When the cheese is cooked, pour the ouzo into the pan and light with a firelighter, standing well, well back as the flames can shoot up. Serve flaming at the table and, when the flames have gone out, squeeze the lemon juice over it and devour!

SERVES 2

2 tablespoons of olive oil

100g/3½ oz of Kasseri per person, cut into palm-sized wedges

2 tablespoons of ouzo

1 lemon

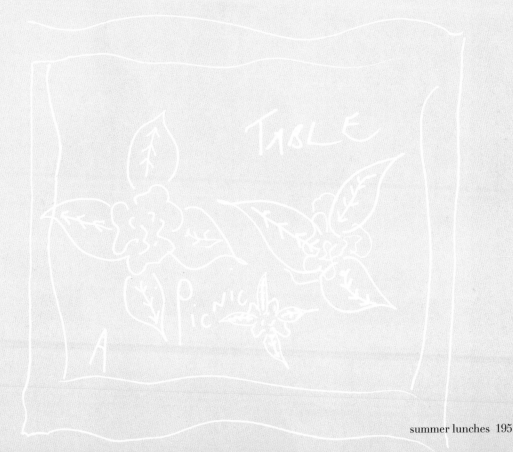

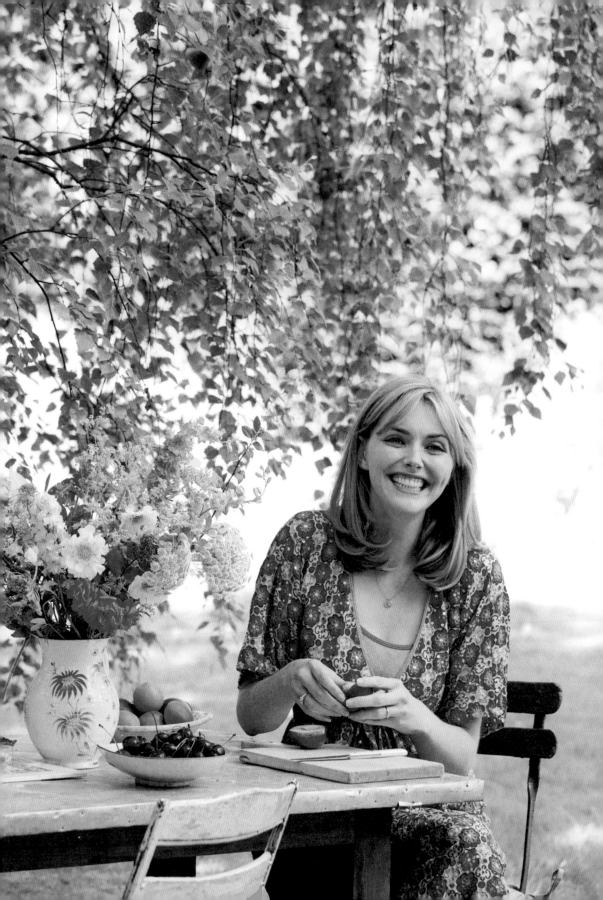

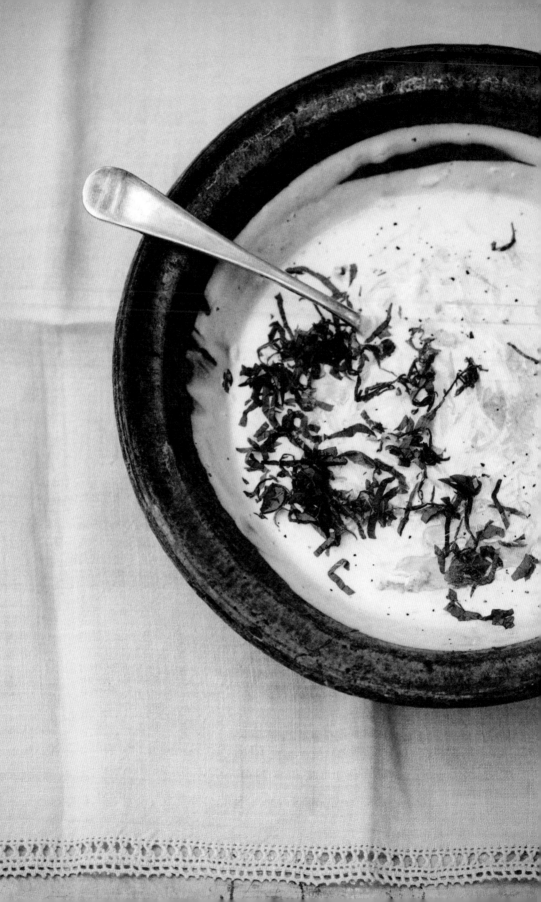

Tzatziki

SERVES 4

1 cucumber
Salt and pepper
250g/1 cup of goat's
    yoghurt or full-fat
    Greek yoghurt
2 cloves of garlic, peeled
    and finely chopped
1 tablespoon of smoky
    olive oil
Juice and zest of ½ a lemon
A handful of fresh mint,
    finely chopped

Peel and deseed the cucumber, and then coarsely grate it. Place it in a colander over the sink and mix it with a few pinches of sea salt. Leave to drain for about 20 minutes or so, and then pat dry with a tea towel.

Put the cucumber in a mixing bowl and add to it the yoghurt and garlic, stirring it all through. Add a tablespoon of olive oil, the zest of half a lemon and a few squeezes of juice. Season it to taste and then add the mint.

Radishes with truffle salt and mint and olive oil

Wash the radishes and finely chop them. Sprinkle them with a pinch of truffle salt, and pour over the olive oil and mint.

SERVES 2–4

A punnet of radishes

A pinch of truffle salt

1 tablespoon of light
    olive oil

A small handful of fresh
    chopped mint

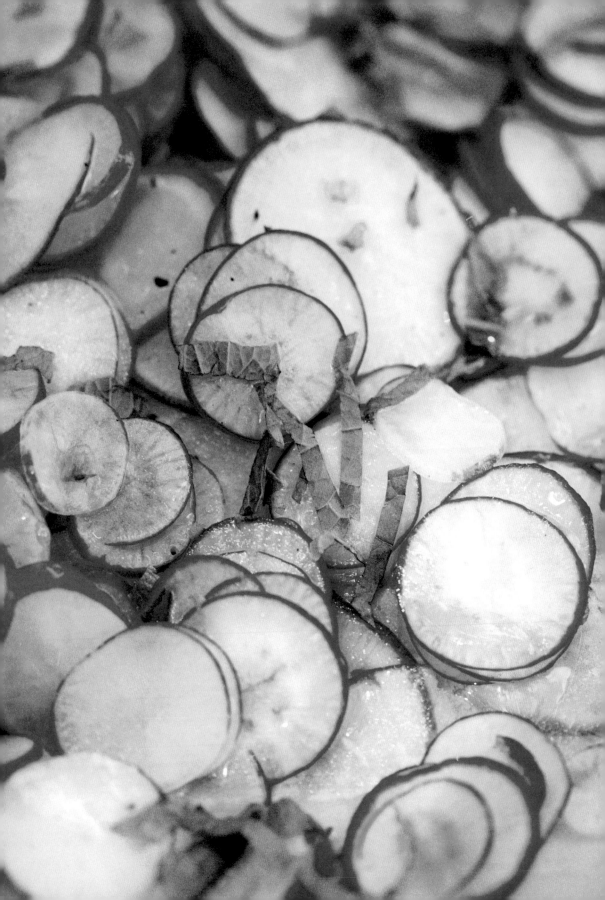

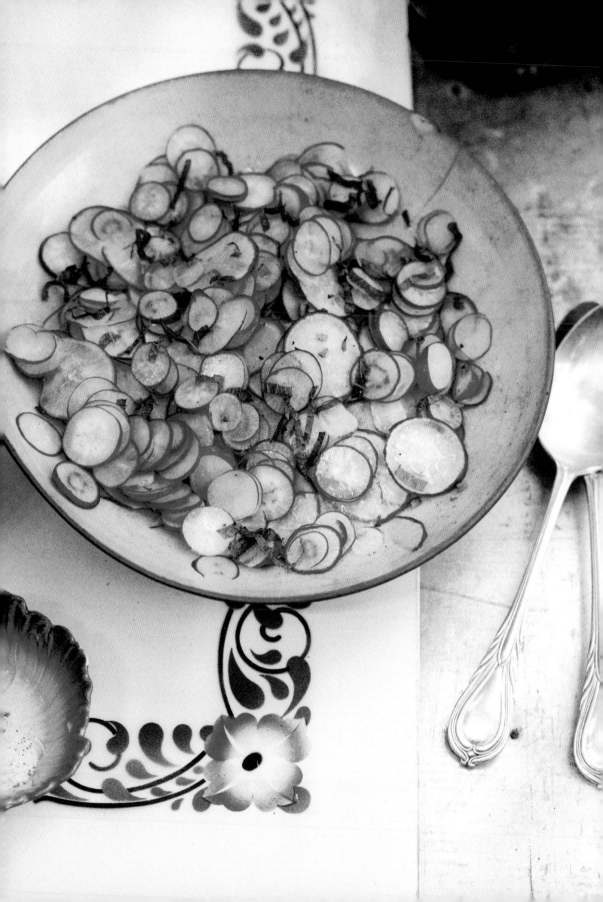

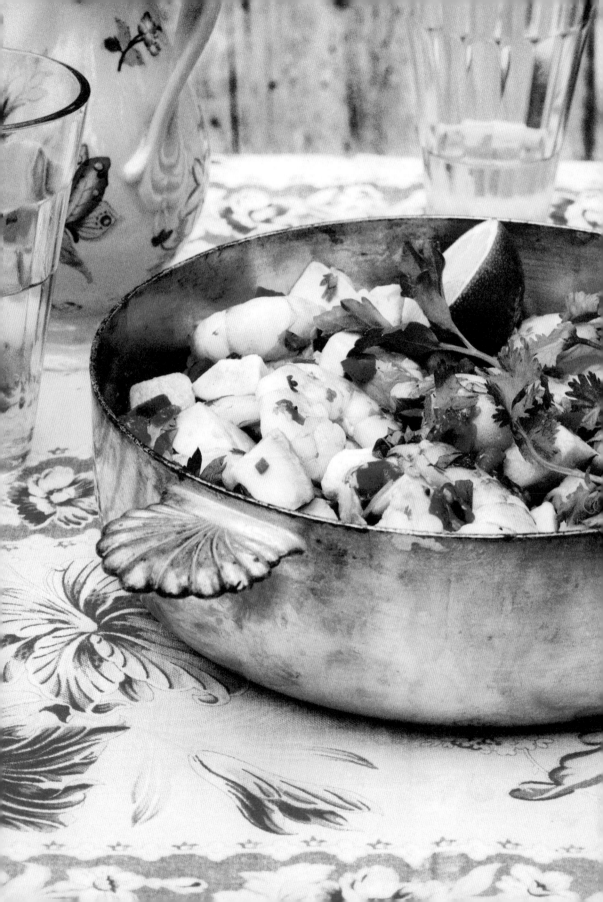

Ceviche with prawns/ shrimp and avocado

Place the prawns/shrimp in a large glass mixing bowl and squeeze the lime juice over them, mixing it all in to make sure they are covered in it. Add the tomatoes, the spring onions/scallions and fresh and dried chilli. Add the herbs. Cover the bowl and refrigerate for at least an hour or so. Stone and chop the avocado and add just before serving so they don't get brown and raddled.

SERVES 4

300g/10oz of peeled raw
   prawns/shrimp
Juice of 3 limes
2 ripe tomatoes, finely
   chopped
2 spring onions/scallions,
   finely chopped
1 red chilli, deseeded and
   finely chopped
A pinch of dried red chilli
   flakes
A small handful of fresh
   chopped parsley
A small handful of
   fresh chopped
   coriander/cilantro
2 ripe avocados

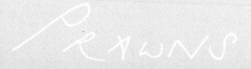

Grilled octopus with potatoes and fagiolini pesto

Grigliata di polpo con patate e pesto di fagiolini
From the kitchen of Antonio Petruzzi

SERVES 4

1 octopus (about 500–
700g/1lb 2oz–1½lb)
4 medium-sized waxy
potatoes
Salt and pepper

For the pesto
200g/7oz of fagiolini
(green beans)
4 tablespoons of extra
virgin olive oil
1 clove of garlic, peeled
Salt and pepper
A small handful of
fresh mint

Cook the octopus in boiling water for approximately 1 hour and a half. In another pan, boil the potatoes for about 15 to 20 minutes, leaving them al dente, then peel them.

Prepare the pesto with the fagiolini beans – it is best to steam them for 5 to 8 minutes so they don't lose their colour. Mix the beans with the oil, garlic, salt and pepper and, at the end, add the mint.

Pull the tentacles from the octopus body and remove anything you find inside the body, including the plastic-like quill. Cut the head off the tentacles and take out the bony beak if still attached. Cut the octopus body and the tentacles into pieces and season with salt and pepper to taste. Preheat the grill or griddle pan to hot and grill for a few minutes. Keep the octopus warm while you then grill the already-sliced potatoes.

Place the grilled potato on a plate, with the octopus nearby, and use a spoon to pour the pesto over the octopus and potato.

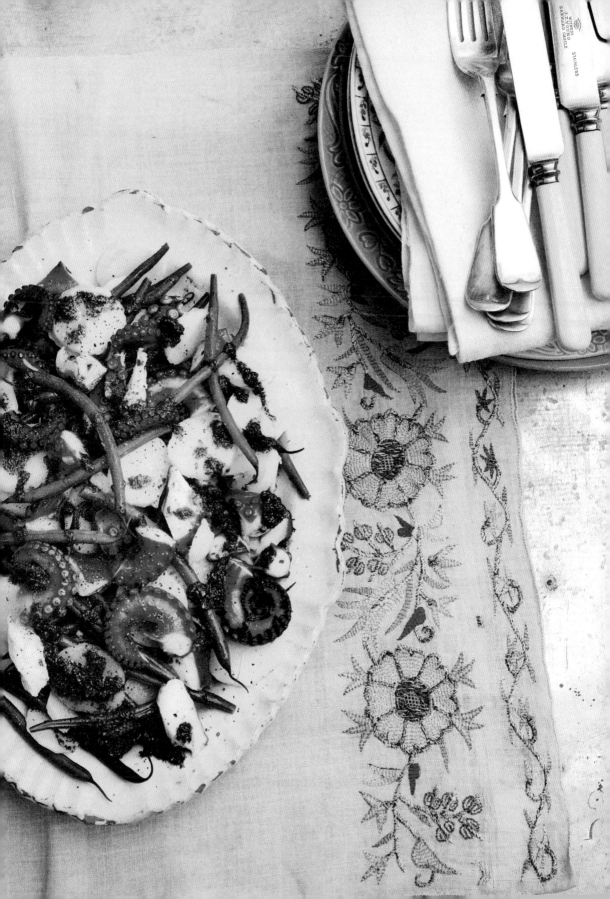

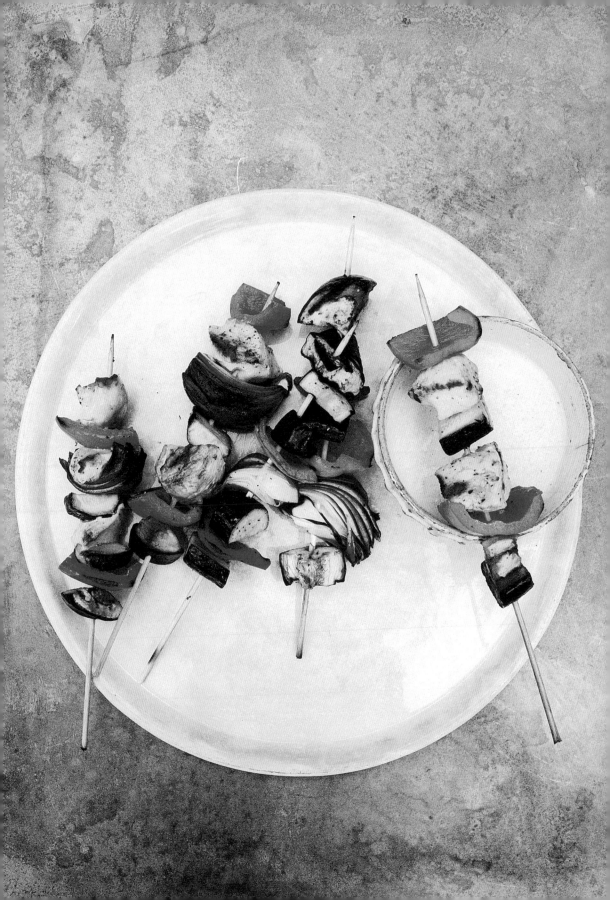

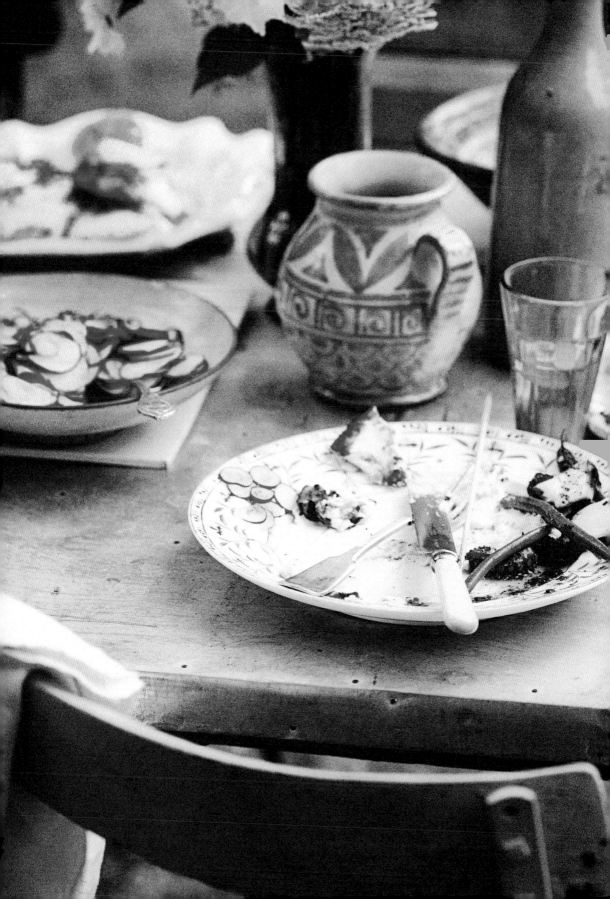

Kebabs

MAKES 8

8 kebab skewers

1 large courgette/zucchini,
cut into rough chunks

1 packet of halloumi
cheese, cut into chunks
(or 250g/9oz of skinless
and boneless chicken
breast, cut into chunks)

1 large red onion, peeled
and cut into chunks

250g/9oz of cherry
tomatoes

For the dressing

250g/1 cup of plain
yoghurt

25g/¼ cup of flaked
almonds

1 clove of garlic, peeled and
roughly chopped

A handful of fresh
coriander/cilantro

A small handful of fresh
mint

Juice of ½ lemon

1 tablespoon of olive oil

If using wooden skewers, soak them for 1 hour in cold water first. Light the barbecue or preheat the grill of the oven.

Assemble the vegetables and cheese on the skewers, alternating courgette/zucchini, chunks of halloumi, onion and whole tomatoes. Leave to one side.

To make the dressing, put all the remaining ingredients in a blender and blitz until smooth. You can now pour this over the skewers before or after cooking them.

Put the skewers on the barbecue or under the grill and cook for about 10 minutes, turning occasionally.

Raw golden beetroot/beets with cayenne and lime

Chop the beetroot/beets as finely as possible into whisper-thin rounds. Assemble onto a really pretty plate. With dry fingers, sprinkle the cayenne pepper on top, then add a healthy squeeze of lime juice and, if you are so moved, a pinch of lime zest.

SERVES 2–3

3 golden beetroot/beets, washed and peeled
½ teaspoon of cayenne pepper
Juice and zest of 1 lime

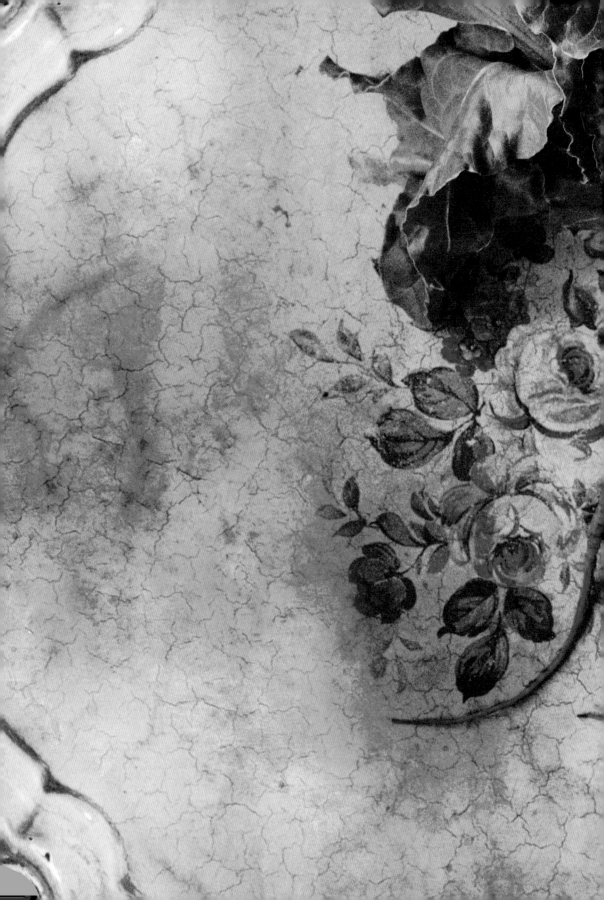

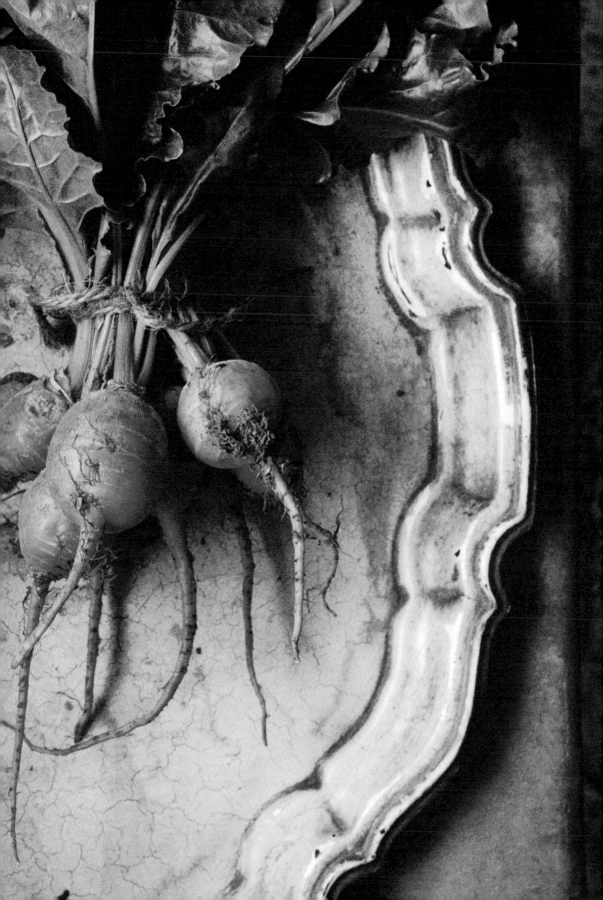

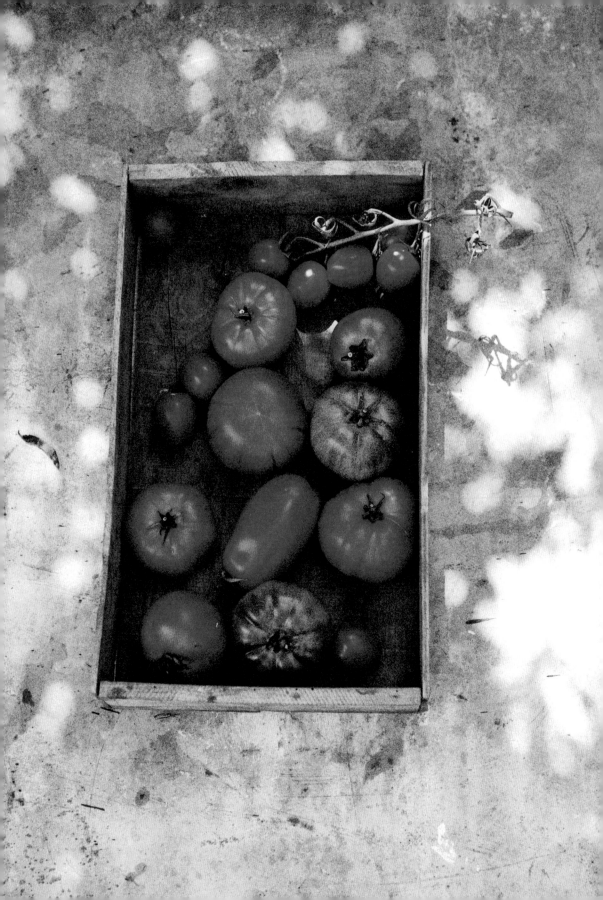

Summer
Suppers

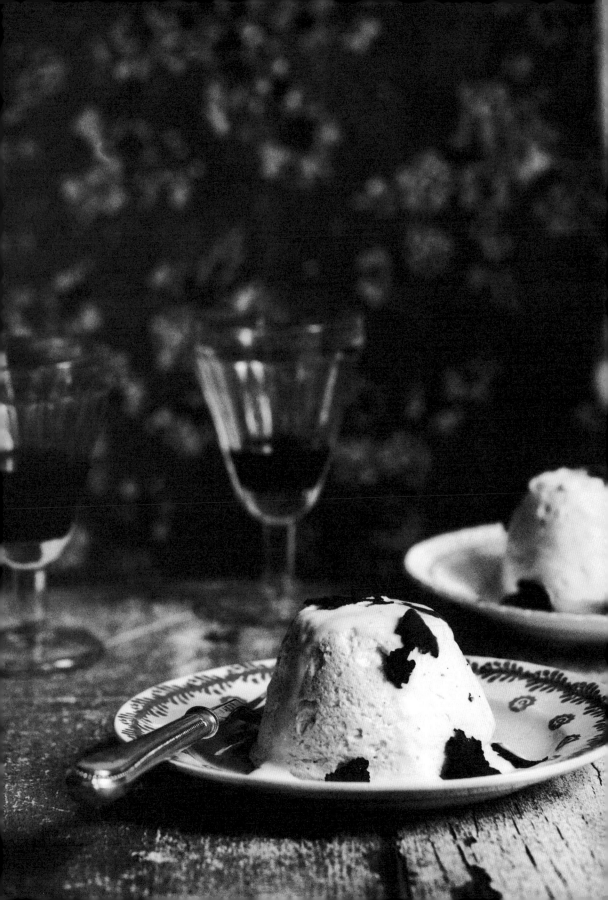

Ricotta tarts with creamy pecorino sauce and shavings of black truffle

Tortino 'soffiato' di ricotta con vellutata di pecorino e scaglie di tartufo nero
Another of Antonio Petruzzi's creations

Preheat the oven to 160°C/140°C fan/Gas 3.

Mix together the ricotta with the egg whites, then add the Parmesan, salt and pepper.

Pour into greased 200ml/7fl oz moulds and bake in the oven for 20 minutes.

In the meantime, heat the pecorino and cream in a bain-marie or a glass bowl over a pan of simmering water, whisking well and adding salt and pepper to taste. Shave the truffle using a vegetable peeler.

Take the tarts out of the oven and place on a plate to serve. Drench the tarts with the creamy sauce and decorate with as much black truffle as you like!

SERVES 4–6

For the tarts
400g/14oz of sheep's
   ricotta cheese
4 egg whites
80g/¾ cup of grated
   Parmesan
Salt and pepper
30g/1oz of black
   truffle

For the creamy sauce
100g/1 cup of grated aged
   pecorino
150ml/generous ½ cup of
   single/light cream
Salt and pepper

Chicken summer stew

SERVES 4–6

3 tablespoons of olive oil

1 small chicken, chopped
   into pieces by your
   butcher

1 onion, peeled and finely
   chopped

2 cloves of garlic, peeled
   and finely chopped

1 teaspoon of ground
   turmeric

250ml/1 cup of white wine

1 cinnamon stick

1 bay leaf

Juice of 1 lemon

250ml/1 cup of chicken
   stock

400g/14oz can of
   chickpeas/garbanzo
   beans, cooked and
   drained

25g/¼ cup of pitted black
   olives

A summery staple. Serve with rice or quinoa. It's much better the next day, as most soups and stews tend to be.

Heat 2 tablespoons of the olive oil in a large casserole on the stove top. Add the chicken pieces and brown, cooking for about 10 to 15 minutes to brown evenly. Remove the chicken from the heat and keep to one side. Using the same pan, add a little more oil and sweat the onion and garlic with the turmeric. After a few minutes, pour the wine over, add the cinnamon stick, the bay leaf and the lemon juice, then add the chicken. Cook this for around 30 minutes, pouring in the stock little by little. Stir in the chickpeas/garbanzo beans and the olives after 20 minutes and serve with a wedge of lemon.

Roasted tomato mascarpone soup with basil oil

Roasting the tomatoes first gives an extraordinary creamy depth to this soup. People tend to think you're lying when you say it has no cream. Make them bet money on it and smile as they pay up. This is also good cold with a swirl of Greek yoghurt or crème fraîche and lots of black pepper.

Preheat the oven to 190°C/170°C fan/Gas 5. Place the tomatoes, onion, red (bell) pepper and garlic in a roasting tray; season with salt and pepper, splash with olive oil and sprinkle over the sugar. Roast for around 45 minutes.

Take the tray out of the oven, allow to cool. Then peel the onion and squeeze out the garlic and place the contents into a blender in batches, depending on the size of your blender, and purée until soft and velvety. When you have a soup, pour it into a large saucepan, on a low heat, add another spoonful of olive oil and stir through the mascarpone. Heat for a minute or two.

Wash the blender out, place the basil and a tablespoon of olive oil in there, and blend on high. Put a swirl of this green mix through the soup just before serving.

SERVES 4

1kg/2¼lb of plum
    tomatoes, halved
1 large onion, quartered
1 large red (bell) pepper,
    deseeded and quartered
4 cloves of garlic
Salt and pepper
Olive oil
1 scant teaspoon of dark
    brown sugar
1 tablespoon of
    mascarpone cheese
A handful of fresh basil

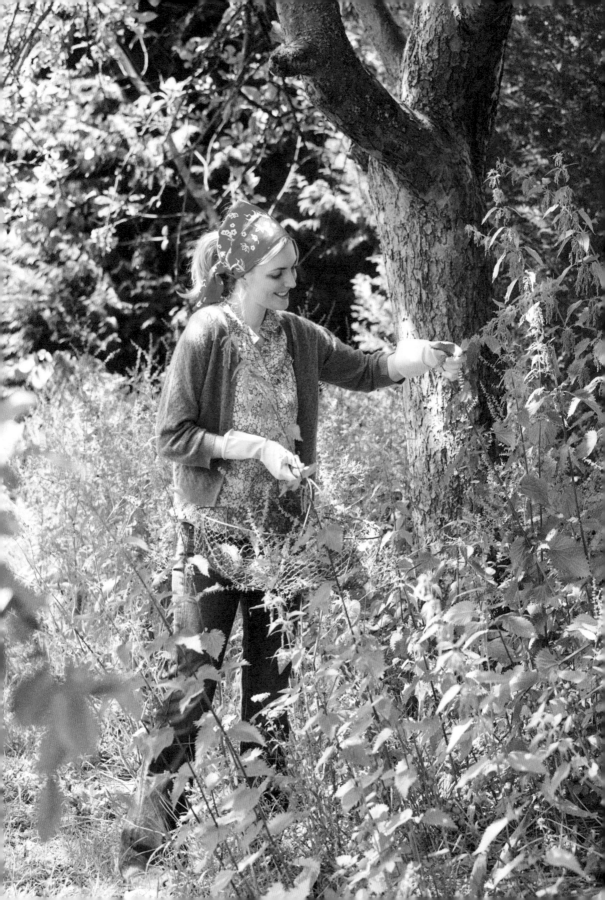

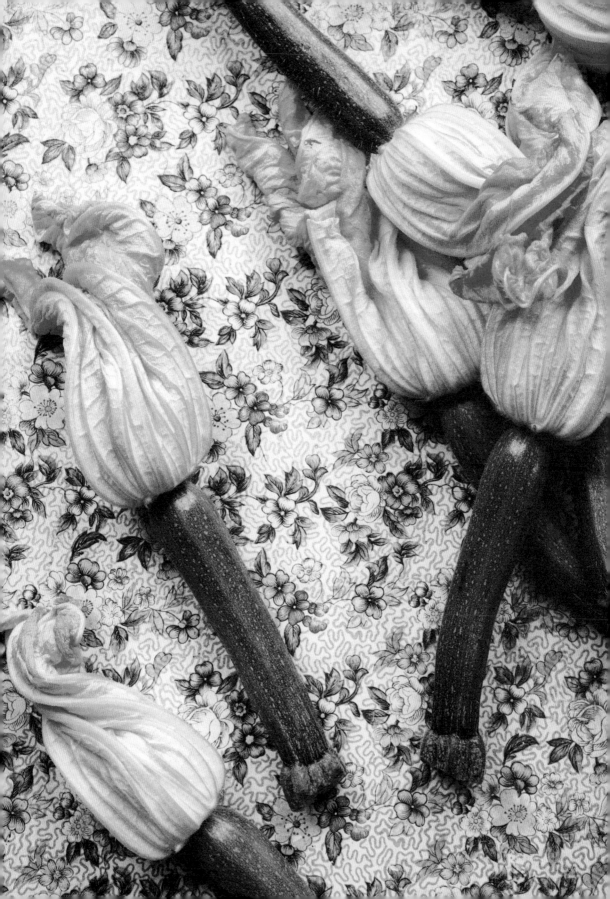

Courgette/ zucchini flower risotto

SERVES 6

8 courgette/zucchini
  flowers with baby
  courgettes/zucchini
  attached
2 tablespoons of olive oil
1 clove of garlic, peeled and
  finely chopped
1 small onion, peeled and
  finely chopped
400g/2 cups of arborio rice
1.5 litres/6½ cups of hot
  stock
60ml/¼ cup of white wine
100g/1 cup of grated
  Parmesan, plus extra for
  serving
Salt and pepper
1 handful of fresh chopped
  basil

There is something hopelessly cheerful about courgette flowers, and they are sweetly adaptable fellows too.

Detach the flowers from the courgettes/zucchini, remove the stamens and gently wipe the flowers clean. Slice the baby courgettes/zucchini into thin rounds.

In a large risotto pan, heat the olive oil and fry the garlic and onion until softened. Add the flowers and stir in for a minute. Put in the rice and coat with the oil, stirring for a minute or so. Pour on a ladleful of stock and stir until it has been absorbed. Repeat this process for about 15 minutes, and then add the baby courgette/zucchini rounds and stir through. Add the white wine, stirring all the while. Cook for another 5 minutes and take off the heat, adding the Parmesan to taste. Season and serve in low bowls with a drizzle of olive oil, some more grated Parmesan and the chopped basil.

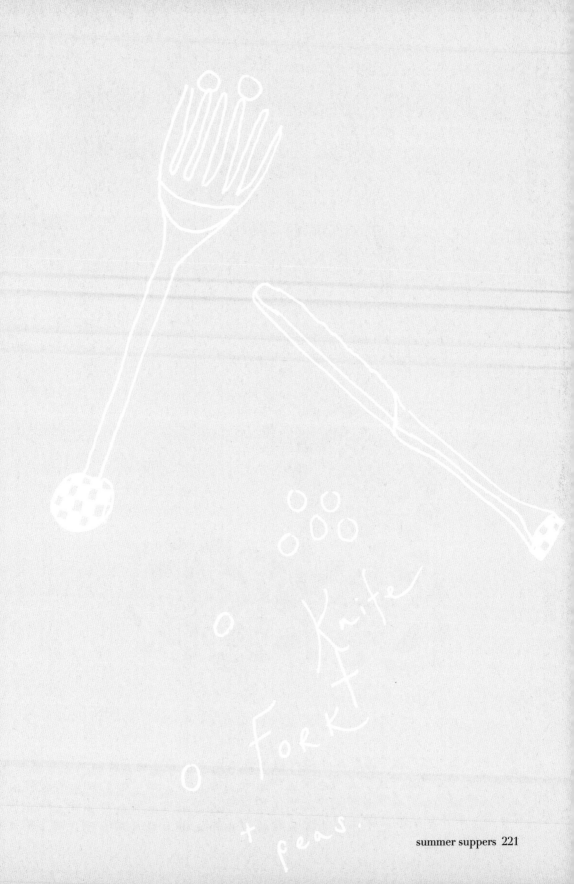

Knife

o Fork

+ peas.

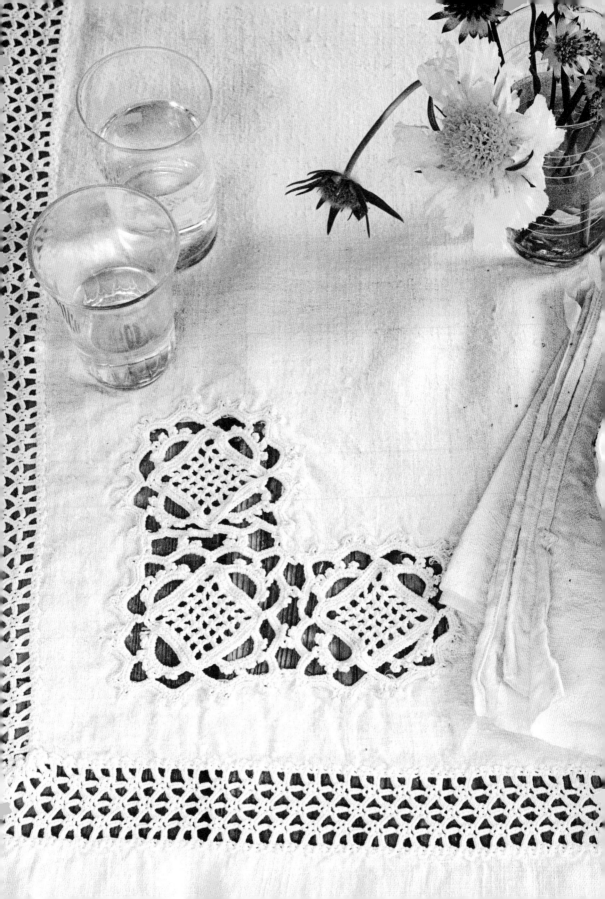

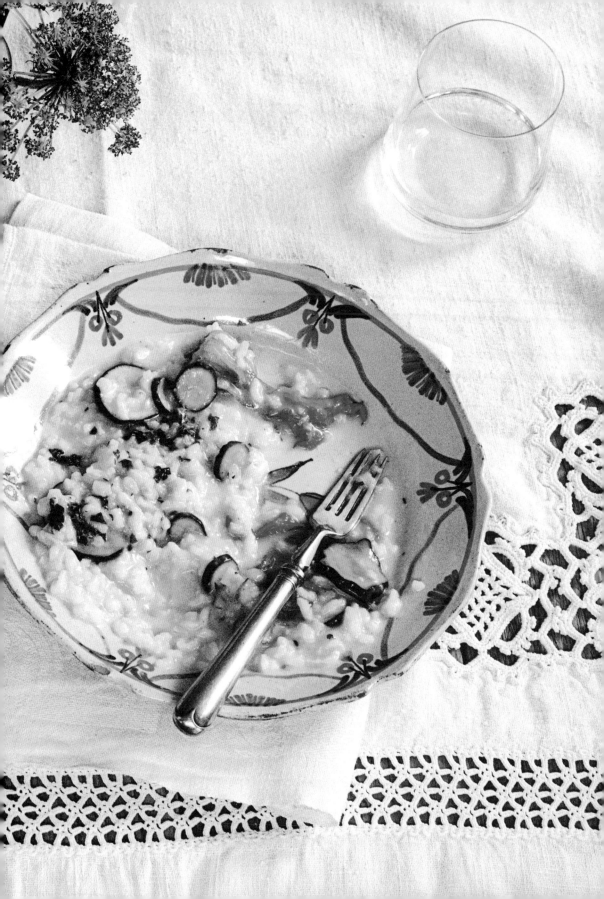

Miso black Colin

SERVES 4

For the marinade
150g/5oz of sweet miso
    paste
2 tablespoons of sake
2 tablespoons of mirin
1 tablespoon of dark brown
    sugar
1 teaspoon of tamari
    (wheat-free soy sauce)

4 pollack fillets, about
    200g/7oz each

Amongst many fish whose names are familiar to us, supplies of cod are being overfished and depleted, which is a cause for very real concern. This is a fact. There are many other fish similar in taste and texture to cod that are sustainable and which you can eat with a clear conscience (for a full list, check the Marine Stewardship Council website). One of these is the pollack. An English supermarket, obviously fearing that the public would be turned off by the name pollack, which seems to me to be a perfectly reasonable name, chose to rechristen the fish a Colin, (the French name for Hake). Yes. So here is a recipe for Miso Black Colin, and imagine the posh diners at Nobu ordering one of those please.

Put all of the marinade ingredients into a saucepan and heat over a medium flame, stirring until all the sugar has melted. Bring to the boil, stir, and take off the heat. Leave to the side until totally cooled.

Wash and dry the fish. The next step is up to you, but I tend to put the marinade into a couple of Ziploc bags, put two fish fillets in each, shake them up to make sure the fish is saturated with the miso, then leave in the fridge overnight. You can also just put the fillets in a shallow dish, pour the marinade on top and leave, covered, in the fridge for a few hours, but the overnight magic is worth it. The fish takes about 6 minutes to cook. Preheat the grill so that it's searing hot and put the fish on a grill pan, pouring any excess marinade on the top. I'd suggest about 3 minutes on each side, serving it with some rice and a salad of cucumbers and shredded spring onions/scallions.

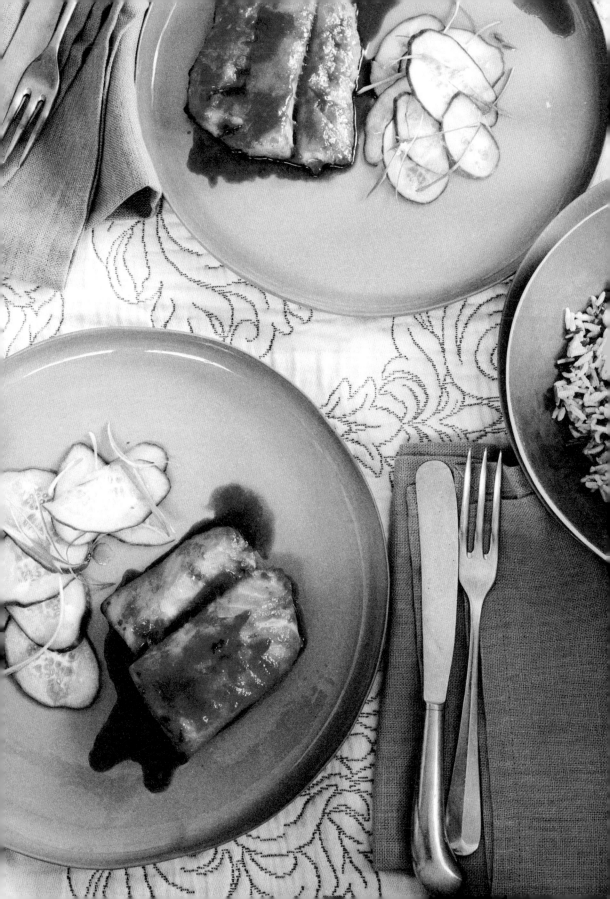

Hangman's Suppers

What do people choose to eat when their number is up? It's a subject I have always been fascinated by. Perhaps unsurprisingly, comfort food, for the most part. In parts of the US where the death penalty is continued, the correctional facility websites provide a macabre insight by listing the last supper wishes of the condemned. They are testimony to childhoods bygone, straight out of a fifties sitcom: fried chicken, grilled cheese on toast, brisket, hamburgers, spare ribs, onion rings and biscuits, mashed potatoes, pecan pie and cheesecake, malted milkshakes and vanilla ice cream. Sweets creep in too – Jolly Ranchers and chocolate bars abound. Though thoroughly limited by their circumstance and place of incarceration, the prisoners are given one last flight in culinary geography. The list dips from the Iowan-corn fed to Tex Mex – refried beans and enchiladas, quesadillas and stuffed peppers – to the pungent memory of a mother's pepperpot stew in the Caribbean, served with a side of ackee and salt fish. Mercifully, an imagined last supper is a hell of a lot easier to get your head around. Chefs are always a good lot to plumb on the topic because they spend a great deal of time thinking about what they're going to eat next, or in this case, last. Once again, the food of childhood seems to win hands down, with Gordon Ramsay, April Bloomfield and Heston Blumenthal all plumping for roast beef and potatoes; Nigella, a lemon roast chicken with creamed spinach, peas à la Française, fennel salad, roast potatoes, chips AND mashed potatoes (I love her); Jamie Oliver, spaghetti and, for pudding, a creamy rice one; and for Raymond Blanc, a shoulder of wild boar steeped in a red wine herby jus, à la Maman. There was a lot of talk of cheese for pudding too. Hugh Fearnley-Whittingstall is adamant his last supper is to be a breakfast, and it is splendidly specific. Scrambled eggs on Granary toast with bacon (streaky, nice and crisp, but not cremated with the rind still on) and mushrooms fried in the bacon fat. All washed down with several strong cups of tea (milk and one sugar).

'I'd have to cook it myself.' he says, 'And make the tea too. After that, I'd have a crisp, tart apple, ideally an Ashmead's Kernel.'

I vacillate with mine. Sometimes it's achingly simple – a poached egg on toast with some pan-fried wild mushrooms on the side, mixed in perhaps with a little butter and some tarragon, garlic and parsley; or a summer pea soup, with a swirl of mint and crème fraîche. Other times, it's the thing that would finish me off before anyone else could. A hearty French onion soup laden with Gruyère and bread, followed by a risotto perfumed with truffles, or a crispy skate wing with some potatoes dauphinoise. Pudding would have to be chocolate, the more molten the better – River Café's Chocolate Nemesis maybe, or a chocolate pot with some brandied cherries lurking in the bottom. At the moment though, written on a rainy day, I think it would be a mound of buttery mashed potatoes with some smoked haddock and a soft poached egg on top, covered in a creamy mustard sauce. But there's also kedgeree, or a thin-crust pizza, charred and sweet with a pool of mozzarella and some fiery chilli oil, or a peanut butter chocolate milkshake. You see the dilemma. Then I remember Café Anglais in Paddington, home to some of the finest food in England. The anchovy and Parmesan custard is the best comfort food, but with none of the stodgy predictability of comfort food. It is rich and grown-up, mysteriously puddingy. It is so good it makes me feel shy. Clever Rowley Leigh.

I think Dustin Hoffman came up with the best back-to-basics hangman's supper ever: mother's milk. 'Might as well go out as you came in.' he mused, in gravel tones.

Rowley Leigh's Parmesan custard with anchovy toast and a herb salad (all mine)

Preheat the oven to 150°C/130°C fan/Gas 2.

Roughly chop the dill and mint and mix in with the rocket/arugula. Dress with your fingers.

Mix the cream, milk and all but a tablespoon of the cheese in a bowl and warm gently over a pan of boiling water until the cheese has melted. Allow to cool completely before whisking in the egg yolks, salt, finely milled white pepper and a little cayenne. Lightly butter eight china moulds (80ml/⅓ cup capacity) and pour in the mixture. Place the moulds in a pan of boiling water, cover with buttered paper and bake in the oven for 15 minutes or until the mixture has just set. Mash the anchovies and butter to a smooth paste and spread over four of the slices of bread. Cover with the remaining bread and toast in a sandwich maker or 'panini' machine.

Sprinkle the remaining Parmesan over the warm custards and brown gently under a hot grill. Cut the toasted anchovy sandwiches into little fingers and serve alongside the custards with the herb salad.

SERVES 4 AS A MAIN OR 8 AS A STARTER

For the herb salad
A handful of fresh dill
A handful of fresh mint
A handful of rocket/arugula
1 tablespoon of olive oil
A squeeze of lemon juice

For the Parmesan custards
300ml/1¼ cups of single/light cream
300ml/1¼ cups of milk
100g/1 cup of finely grated Parmesan
4 egg yolks
Salt and white pepper
Cayenne pepper

For the anchovy toasts
12 anchovy fillets
50g/½ stick of unsalted butter
8 very thin slices of pain de campagne

Broad bean/fava risotto

SERVES 6

300g/2 cups of podded
  fresh or frozen
  broad/fava beans
1 tablespoon of olive oil
25g/¼ stick of butter
1 small onion, peeled and
  finely chopped
1 clove of garlic, peeled and
  finely chopped
400g/2 cups of
  Arborio rice
125ml/½ cup of white wine
1.2 litres/5 cups of hot
  vegetable or chicken
  stock
100g/2 cups of baby
  spinach
100g/1 cup of pecorino,
  grated, plus extra for
  serving

There is something lovely and lulling about shelling broad beans at the kitchen table, stealing a few as you go. Another one of my favourite summer things is broad beans with sea salt, a hunk of pecorino and some chopped mint and olive oil. It is total perfection on its own. I guess this risotto is the graduation of that.

Bring a pan of salted water to the boil and cook the broad/fava beans for 5 to 6 minutes. Drain and tip the beans into a bowl of cold water. Drain again, then pop the beans out of their skins and set aside.

In a heavy-bottomed pan, heat the olive oil and butter on a lowish heat. Sweat the onion for a few minutes until translucent, then add the garlic, taking care it doesn't burn. Add the rice to the pan, giving it a good stir. Pour in the wine and cook until it's all been absorbed. Breathe.

Add the stock, ladle by ladle, stirring well between each addition and topping up only when the last ladle has been absorbed. The trick to risotto is surrendering to the stirring, finding a calm in it. When the stock is used up, you're about there; it normally takes around 20 minutes. A few minutes before this point, stir in the broad/fava beans, spinach and pecorino to taste. Plate in low bowls, with a bit of pecorino.

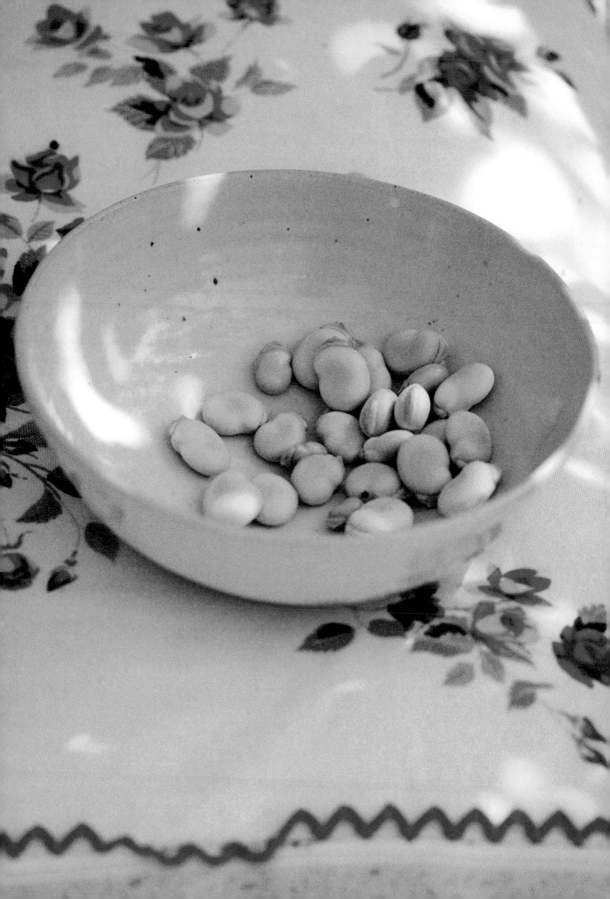

Puddings

Marbled rose petal ice cream

Chocolate meringue biscuits

Pineapple and mint granita

Poached winter fruits with crème anglaise

Uncle's chocolate soufflé with brandied cherries

Earl Grey and lavender ice cream

Rice pudding cake

Almost mother-in-law cake

Panettone bread-and-butter pudding

Coconut sorbet

Ruby Frais strawberry semifreddo

Armagnac apricot pannacotta

Christmas sugar plum syllabubby mess

Roses

I first went to India when I was twelve. We stayed in an ashram surrounded by mountains with pale pink stone floors and mango trees whose branches trailed the ground like old ladies' fingers. I loved everything about it. The dawn call to prayer, beating a solitary wail against the thick morning air; the sweet lassi that you had mid morning to keep you going, and at lunch time; the trays piled high with rice, dhal and chapati. I loved the statues that peppered the landscape, all the gods from Hindu scriptures, amongst them cheeky Hanuman the monkey god and Ganesh the elephant with the little mouse who sat watchfully at his feet. My favourite was Lakshmi, the goddess of abundance, whose beauty and benevolence was protected from the elements by the stone shell in which she sat.

In the evening, we children were allowed to walk down the dirt road into the local village, where moon-eyed garlanded cows wandered in and out of people's yards and bats swooped so low that they could get caught in your hair if it was long enough. I wore mine up in a French plait because I had heard the shriek of the tall thirteen-year-old whose mother had spent hours armed with scissors and an iron will as she tried to release the clumsy bat from her daughter's thick nest of curls. The thought of those wings beating against my head made me shiver, and I stooped on these twilight walks, hair tight and unwelcoming.

The village had an unmistakable smell to it: bonfires, incense, raw gasoline, jasmine, dung and rosewater. It was heady and alien and crept around you like smoke. We passed the fishermen on the bridge and the dhobi washer man's shop, where if you took your underclothes they laughed at you, and we walked by the sadhu, who had rheumy eyes and stood ruler straight, never seeming to move.

The sweet stall was run by a woman whose generous flesh fell over the folds of her tight orange sari, with a thick black coil of hair that any bat would be fool to invade. She smiled when she saw our greedy eyes and said, 'Good evening, good evening.'

'Good evening Ma!' We chorused, grubby rupee notes unfurling from hot hands.

Her wares sat in paper cases stained with ghee. Carrot and pistachio halva and coconut burfi, and below, swimming in stainless steel bowls, were my very own downfall, the sloppy milk-fed nursery puddings. The celestial rasmalai in a sweet wave of condensed milk, fat orange dumplings bobbing in a pure sugar syrup, Gulab jamun to the uninitiated. The other marvel was a pale concoction seemingly dreamed up by the deities, vermicelli kheer, which sang of cardamom, rosewater and almonds.

A pudding that actually tasted of roses – what a thing!

It wasn't until years later when I was an adult with my own kitchen that I tried to mimic the rosy alchemy that I tasted in India. Rather than using rosewater, I experimented with the real thing – some fat, blowsy pink tea roses in the height of their bloom. Because English summers are often so horribly unpredictable, I suggest making the following and putting it in the freezer at the ready for one of those of those rare halcyon Indian summer nights, where the garden is ripe, voluptuous and welcoming. And if you don't have a garden, you can simply conjure up some tea lights, throw open the windows and put a thick picnic rug on the floor. To enhance the mood further, a soundtrack of Bhangra or, for the more mellow, the sitar strains of Ravi Shankar.

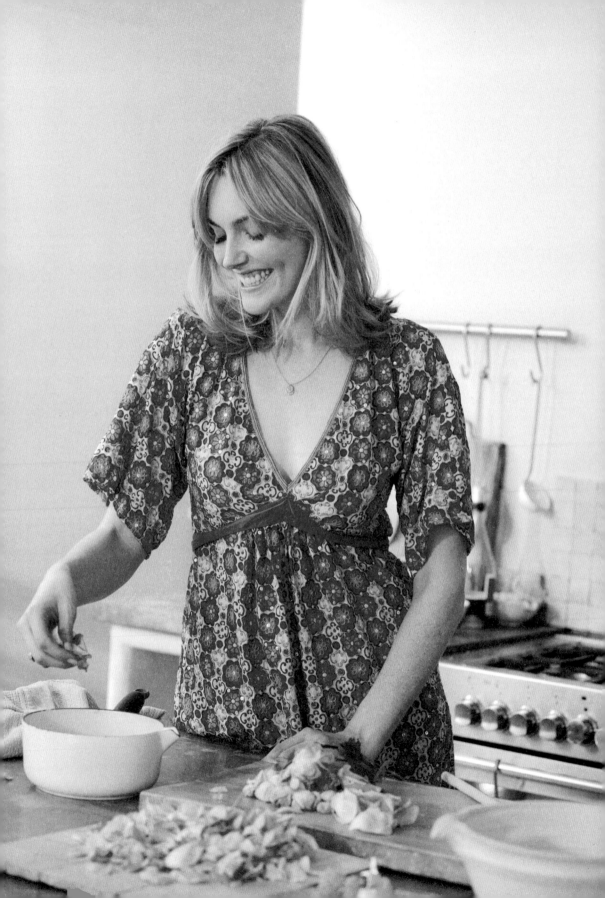

Marbled rose petal ice cream

Pour the sparkling rosé and sugar in a saucepan on a low heat. Add the rose petals and keep on stirring until the sugar has dissolved. Using a slotted spoon, remove three-quarters of the rose petals and set aside. Carry on reducing the sugar syrup on a medium heat until thick and syrupy. Allow the mix to cool.

In a separate mixing bowl, cream the sugar and egg yolks until pale in colour, and keep to the side.

In a saucepan, heat the milk and cream until they reach boiling point. Remove from the stove. Whisking the whole time, temper the egg mixture and bring it up to the same temperature as the cream by adding the milk and cream mixture slowly. Add the remaining rose petals. Before churning, keep to one side to cool and then remove the petals.

Pour the custard into your ice-cream maker with half of the rose petal jam and churn as per the instructions. If you do not have an ice-cream maker, you can do the following for all the ice cream recipes. Freeze the mixture in a plastic container for 2 hours. Remove from the freezer, pour into a blender and whiz for a minute or two. Pour back into the container. Freeze for another 2 hours, then serve. Take the ice cream out of the machine or container and swirl the remaining petal jam roughly through the ice cream to make a marbled pink surface. Place in the freezer to set.

SERVES 4

For the rose petal jam
500ml/2 cups of sparkling
   rosé
40g/¼ cup of
   caster/superfine sugar
20g/¾oz fragrant rose
   petals, washed

125g/½ cup of
   caster/superfine sugar
8 egg yolks
500ml/2 cups of milk
500ml/2 cups of
   double/heavy cream

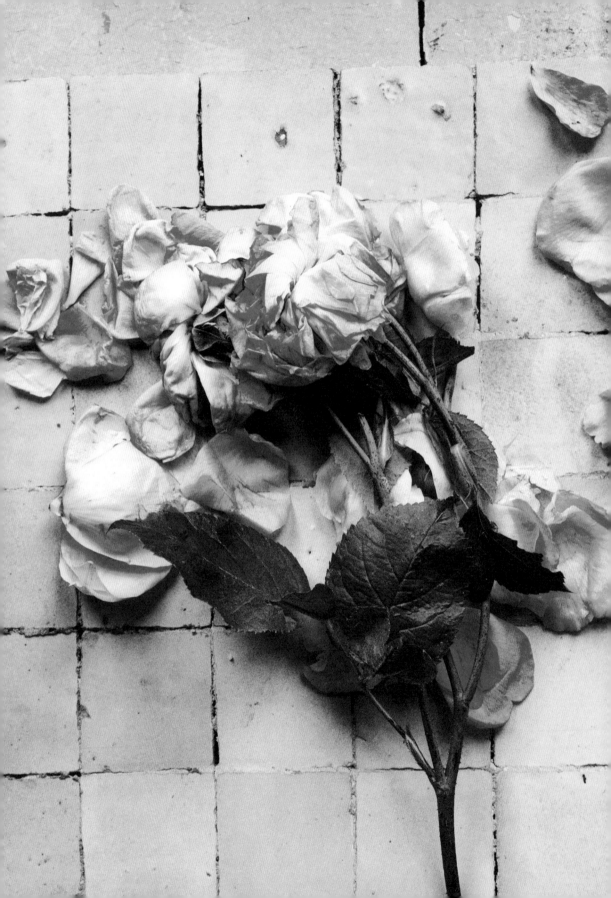

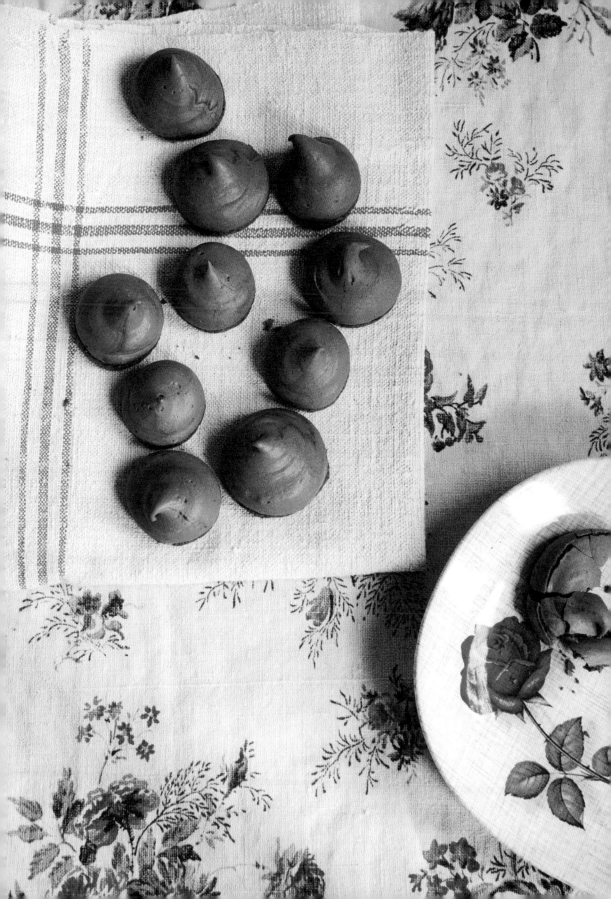

Chocolate meringue biscuits

MAKES ROUGHLY 15 BISCUITS

3 large egg whites
A pinch of cream of tartar
Double the eggs' weight in
  caster/superfine sugar
200g/7oz of dark
  chocolate, broken up
60g/½ cup of good-quality
  cocoa
Extra cocoa, to dust

I love chocolate meringue, hopefully with some sorbet, ice cream or bashed-up raspberries and cream involved. These are glossy and easy and very good.

Preheat the oven to its lowest setting.

In a very clean bowl, whisk the egg whites until frothy and then add the cream of tartar. Carry on whisking the whites until they are at the stiff peaky stage and then, very slowly, add the sugar, a tablespoon at a time.

In a bain-marie, or a heatproof bowl over a pan of boiling water, melt the chocolate and sift the cocoa into the mix. When the chocolate is smooth and glossy, slowly fold into the glossy meringue mixture.

Pipe or spoon the chocolate meringue mixture onto a baking tray lined with non-stick baking/parchment paper. Place in the oven for 45 to 55 minutes. When the meringues have cooled, dust with the extra cocoa.

Pineapple and mint granita

During my first trimester of pregnancy I craved pineapple, particularly in this form. I dreamt of it, and carried whole pineapples up to bed with me, hacking into them in the night like some rotund jungle explorer. There is something about the sweet, refreshing coolness of pineapple mixed with the mint that banishes morning sickness, and for that I am thankful.

SERVES 4–6

2 pineapples, skin removed
and cut into chunks
2 sprigs of fresh mint
Agave syrup or sugar, to
sweeten (optional)

Place the pineapple chunks in a food processor and whiz until you have mostly juice. Strain the pineapple juice through a fine sieve. This makes around 500ml/2 cups of juice. You can use bought pineapple juice if you like, but fresh pineapple is pretty spectacular.

In a heatproof bowl, blanch the mint sprigs with a little boiling water and then remove and run immediately under ice-cold water. Chop the mint finely and stir into the strained pineapple juice. Taste and add agave or sugar if you think you should.

Freeze in a shallow metal container for around 2 hours. Check on it and use a fork to break up what should be shards of icy pineapple mixture. Once you've broken it up, refreeze again for a few hours.

Using a fork, shave the crushed pineapple mixture into glasses and serve.

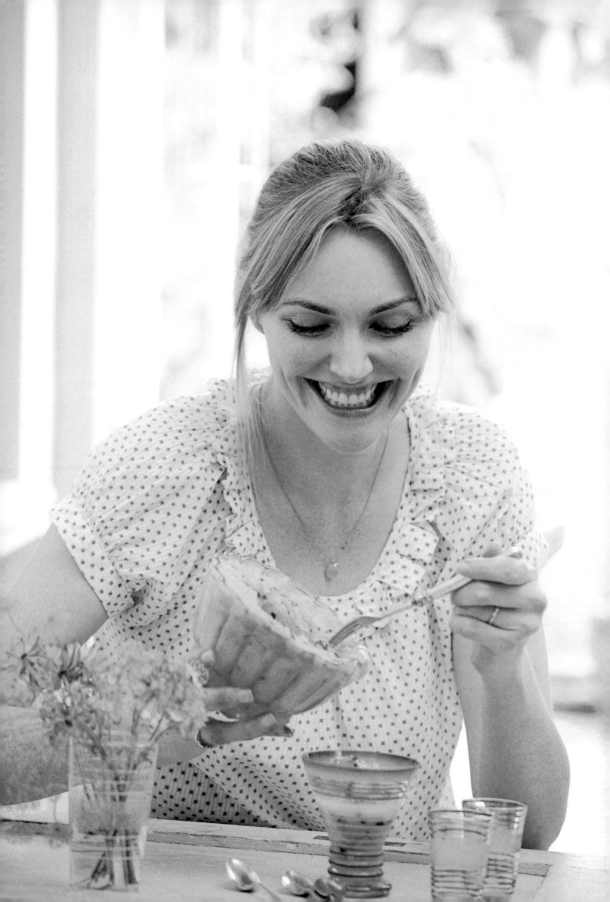

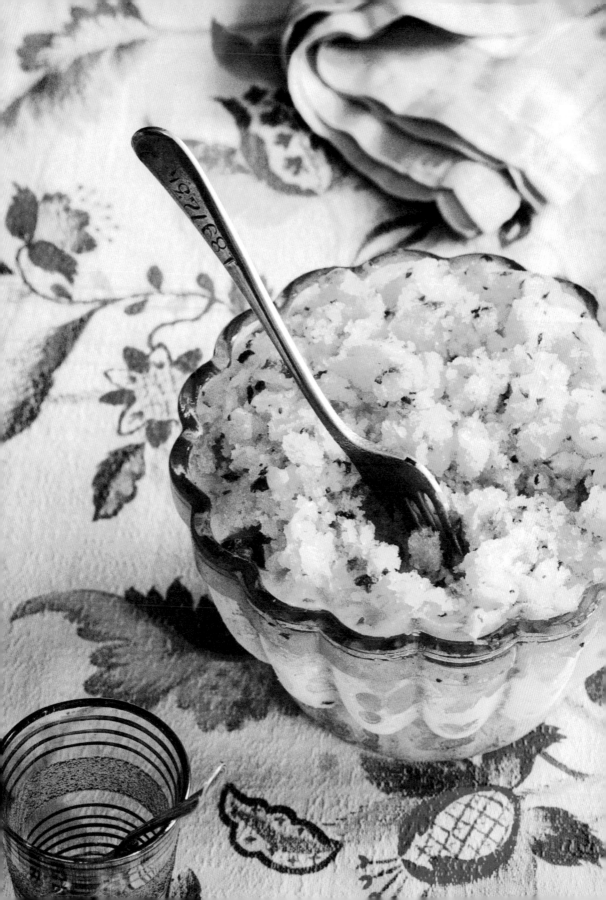

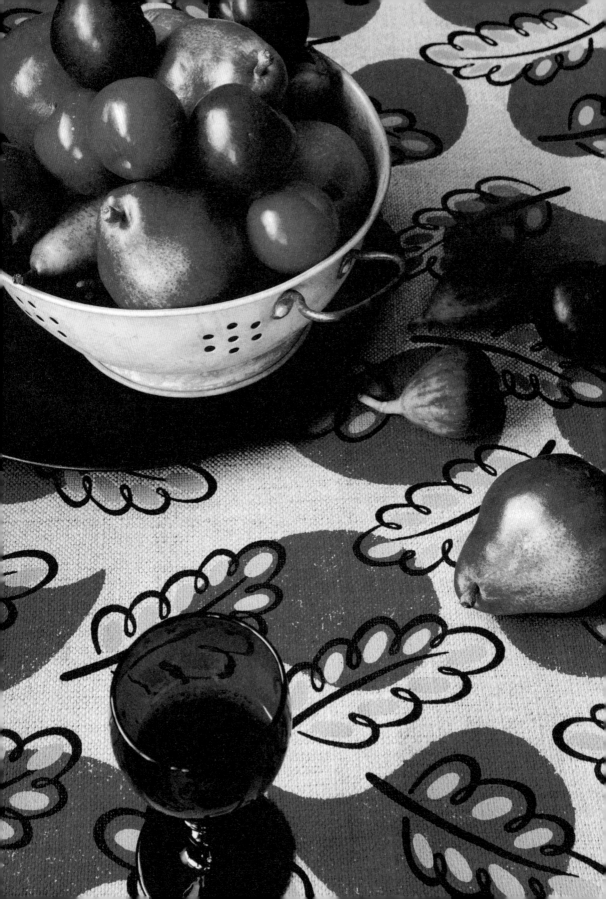

Poached winter fruits with crème anglaise

You could just as well serve this alongside a Christmassy breakfast, and you can totally play around with the fruit you use. It works as a lighter pudding after a hearty meal.

Poach the fruits in a large saucepan with a small amount of water. Start with the quince, poaching for around 8 minutes, and then add the pears and apples and cook for another 10. With 5 minutes to go, add the figs and plums.

In a separate saucepan, mix the wine, sugar, cinnamon, bay, cloves, star anise and orange and bring to the boil. Simmer for around 10 to 15 minutes. When both the fruit and the wine syrup have cooled, pour the syrup over the fruit and leave covered overnight.

Make the crème anglaise shortly before serving. Bring the milk and the vanilla to the boil, take off the heat and allow to infuse. In a heatproof bowl, mix together the egg yolks and the sugar, and place over a saucepan of boiling water. Whisk briskly. Gradually strain the vanilla milk in to the yolks and sugar and continue to stir as it thickens. Take off the heat and serve over your fruit.

SERVES 4

For the fruit

1 quince, peeled, cored and quartered

2 pears, as above

2 apples, as above

2 figs, quartered

2 plums, stoned and quartered

500ml/2 cups of fruity red wine

100g/½ cup of caster/superfine sugar

1 cinnamon stick

1 bay leaf

A few cloves

1 star anise

A few slices of orange

For the crème anglaise

150ml/generous ½ cup of full-fat milk

1 vanilla pod/bean, insides scraped

4 egg yolks

50g/¼ cup of caster/superfine sugar

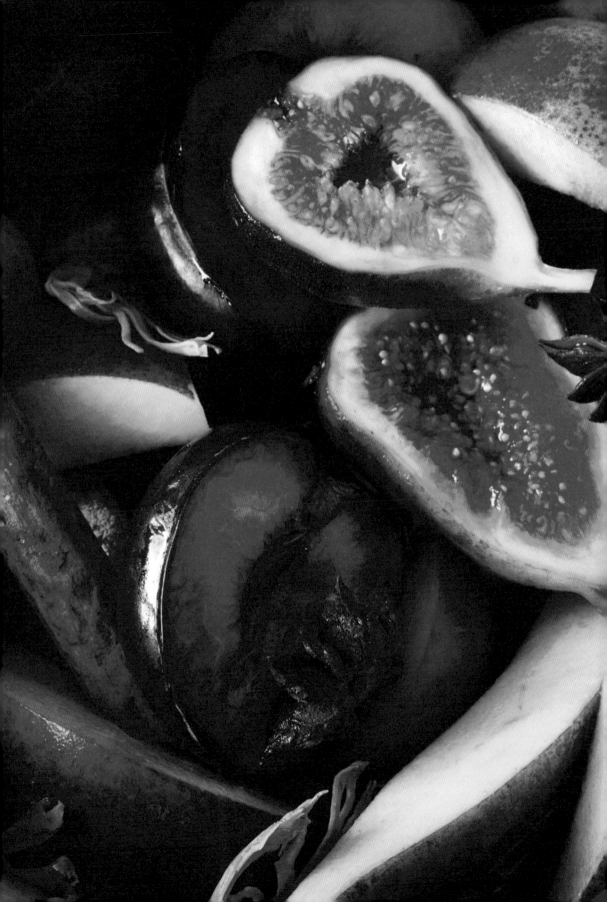

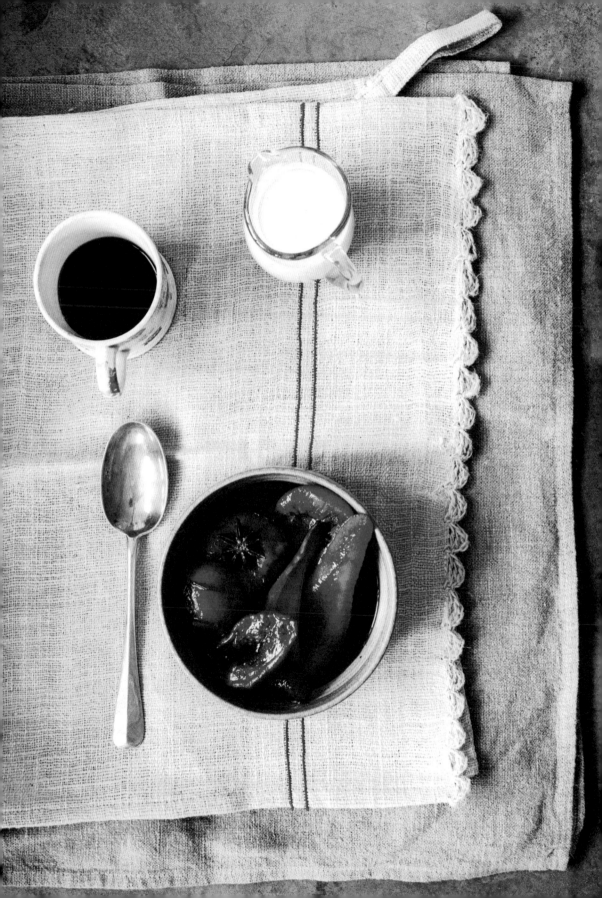

Uncle's chocolate soufflé with brandied cherries

Ned is my littlest brother, who is seventeen. He is divine. At six foot three and still growing, he is not little; he is like a long bean. For some meandering reason, my other brother and sister and I call him 'Uncle'. Whenever we see him, we sing a very annoying Uncle theme song to him to the tune of 'Let's Get Ready to Rumble' and, understandably, it drives him a little insane. I think he may end up a politician. He has always been quite particular when it comes to food. Onions are banished, as is garlic, and mushrooms don't get a look in. He does, however, like chocolate. This chocolate soufflé then is for him, but perhaps without the brandied cherries (which I'm imagining he might be appalled by). His version would probably have ice cream.

Preheat the oven to 150°C/130°C fan/Gas 2.

Using a knob of butter, grease the inside of four ramekins. Place your chocolate in a bain-marie, or a heatproof bowl over a pan of boiling water. Stir the chocolate, so it melts evenly. Keep on a low heat. In a very clean dry bowl, whisk the egg whites. I do this in my KitchenAid as it makes life very easy. When the egg whites are glossy and stiffening, start adding the sugar, bit by bit.

Take your chocolate off the heat and whisk the egg yolks into it. Very gently, add the chocolate to the egg whites. The key is to fold in rather than mix or whisk because you want it to stay as light as a feather. GENTLY fold into the ramekins, smoothing the edges with your thumb, which will help them rise. Place the ramekins on a baking tray, place in the oven and don't you open that door for 20 minutes! Serve immediately.

To distract from soufflé anxiety, make the cherries. In a small saucepan, combine the cherries with the brandy, sugar and water. Cook on a low to medium heat until the cherries are soft and sloppy, but still holding their basic shape. Serve alongside your beauteous soufflés.

SERVES 4

100g/3½oz of really good-
    quality dark chocolate
4 egg whites
50g/¼ cup of golden
    caster/superfine sugar
2 egg yolks

For the brandied cherries
A handful of pitted
    cherries
1 tablespoon of brandy
1 tablespoon of sugar
80ml/⅓ cup of water

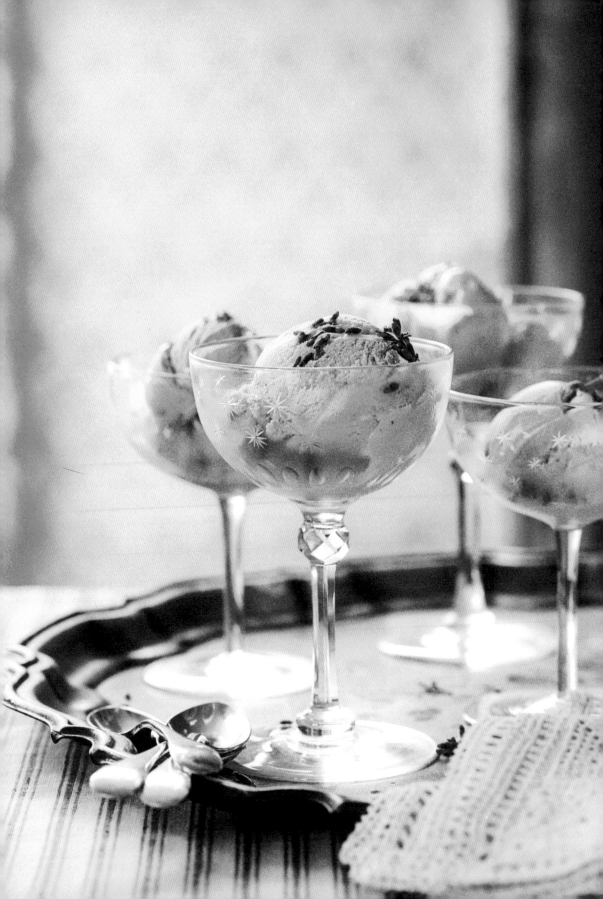

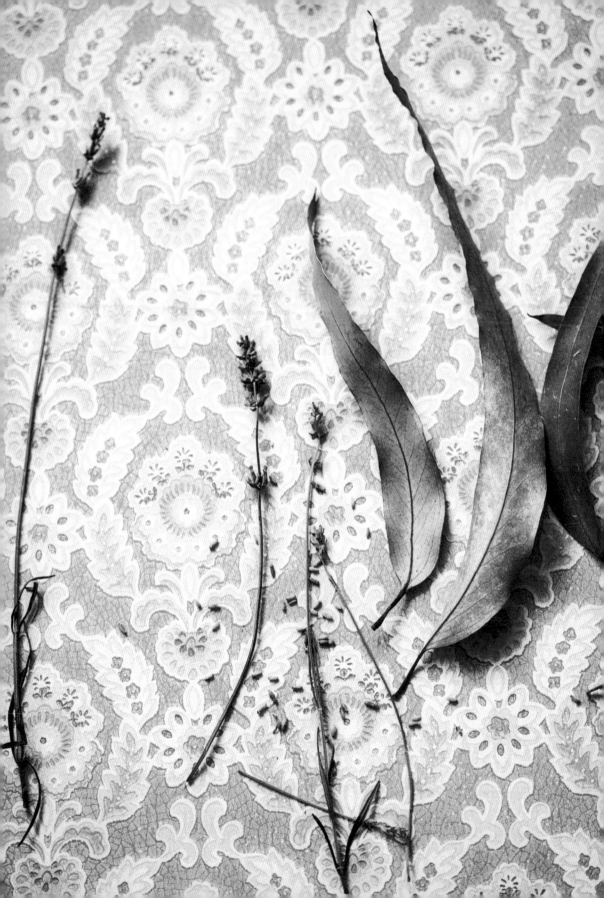

Earl Grey and lavender ice cream

SERVES 4

Muslin bag and string, for
   a bouquet garni
1 tablespoon fresh
   chopped lavender leaves
4 tablespoons Earl Grey
   tea leaves
8 egg yolks
125g/½ cup of
   caster/superfine sugar
500ml/2 cups of
   double/heavy cream
500ml/2 cups of milk

Earl Grey works beautifully with lavender. You can also make a wonderful iced tea using Earl Grey, lavender and a sugar syrup, steeping and leaving in the fridge to cool.

First make your bouquet garni by tying the lavender and Earl Grey tea leaves into the muslin bag. Make sure the string is tightly knotted. Put to one side.

In a mixing bowl, cream the egg yolks and sugar until pale and creamy and keep to one side.

In a heavy-bottomed saucepan, heat the cream, milk and bouquet garni of lavender and tea leaves up until boiling point, and then remove from the stove.

Temper the egg and sugar mixture by slowly adding the infused cream to bring the egg up to the same temperature, whisking all the time. Strain the mixture and then allow it to cool.

Churn in your ice-cream maker as per the instructions. If you do not have an ice-cream maker, freeze the mixture in a plastic container for 2 hours. Remove from the freezer, pour into a blender and whiz for a minute or two. Pour back into the container. Freeze for another 2 hours, then serve.

Rice pudding cake

This is a risotto cake of sorts. It was made for me by an Italian mama in Sorrento, and the recipe was mimed in a clamouring kitchen. I think that it has worked regardless!

Preheat the oven to 160°C/140°C fan/Gas 3.

Into a large saucepan on the stovetop, pour the milk and then add the rice. Add to this the orange zest and cook on a low heat, stirring frequently, until the rice has absorbed all the milk. This should take around 15 minutes. Take the pan off the heat and let it cool.

When the milky rice has cooled, mix in the sugar, eggs, butter, raisins and almonds. Grease a springform tin/pan and sprinkle with half the crushed amaretti biscuits.

Pour the rice mixture into the pan and cook for around 45 minutes. To serve, dust with the remaining crushed amaretti biscuits and orange zest.

SERVES 4

1 litre/4 cups of milk
160g/¾ cup of Arborio rice
Zest of 1 orange
150g/½ cup of caster/superfine sugar
3 eggs
2 tablespoons of butter
50g/¼ cup of raisins
50g/½ cup of flaked almonds
4 tablespoons of crushed amaretti biscuits
Finely grated orange zest, to decorate

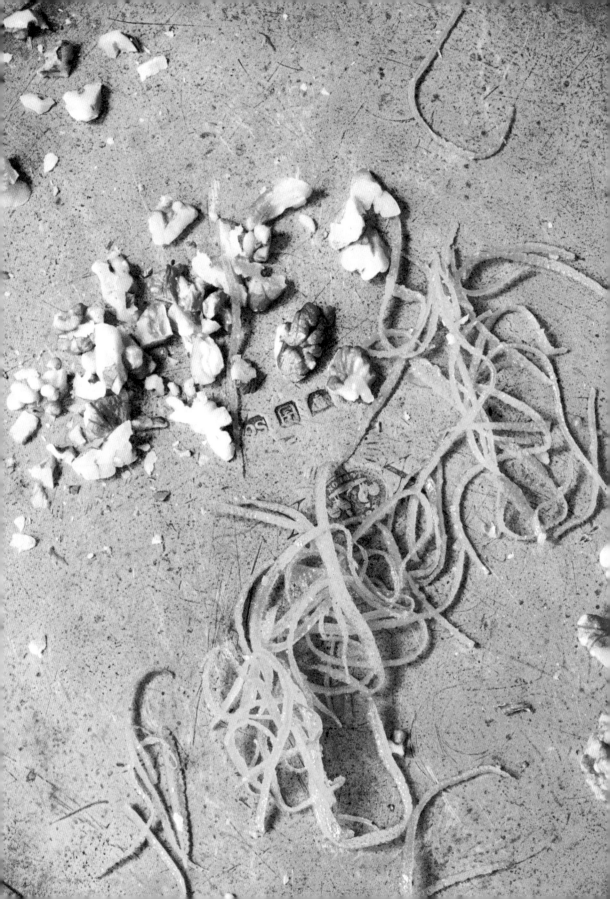

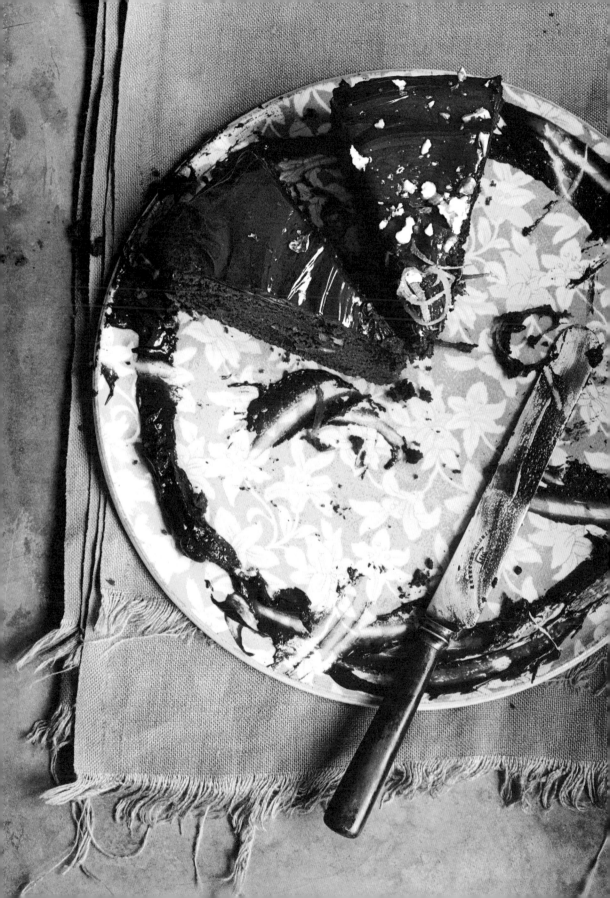

Almost mother-in-law cake

SERVES 4–6

300g/3 sticks of butter,
very soft
500g/2 cups of
caster/superfine sugar
4 eggs
350g/3 cups of plain/all-
purpose flour, sifted
75g/generous ½ cup of
cocoa, sifted
2 teaspoons of baking
powder
2 teaspoons of vanilla
extract
125ml/½ cup of milk, at
room temperature
rather than chilled
125ml/½ cup of boiling
water
Juice and finely grated zest
of 1 orange
120g/1 cup of chopped
walnuts, plus extra to
decorate
Shredded candied orange
zest, to decorate

*For the chocolate
ganache*
250g/9oz good-quality
dark chocolate, chopped
250ml/1 cup of
double/heavy cream

This recipe was sent to me by a reader, called Sabine. It was passed on to her by her 'almost mother-in-law', to whom we are spectacularly grateful. 'Almost weddings' can wax and wane, but chocolate cake is here to stay, and this one, like Sabine who sent it is lovely, the orange and walnuts happy bedfellows.

Preheat the oven to 180°C/160°C fan/Gas 4.

Mix everything (except the extra walnuts and candied orange zest) together, one after another, in the order they are listed. Beat until smooth and pour into a 25-cm/10-inch cake tin/pan lined with baking/parchment paper. Bake for about 1 hour.

To make the icing, place the chocolate in a bain-marie, or a bowl over a pan of boiling water. Stir the chocolate, so it melts evenly. Bring the cream to boiling point in a small pan, and then pour over the chocolate, stirring occasionally until smooth and glossy.

Thickly spread/swirl the icing over the top and sides of the cake with a palette knife or spatula and top with the extra walnuts and candied orange zest.

Panettone bread-and-butter pudding

Bread-and-butter pudding is an English staple; proper nursery food. Panettone makes it a bit more interesting and festive – this is a good one for around Christmas time when you want a hearty, warming pudding.

Preheat the oven to 190°C/170°C fan/Gas 5.

Whisk together the cream, milk and eggs. Slice the vanilla pod/bean in half and scrape the seeds into the egg and cream mixture. Add the caster/superfine sugar and whisk some more.

Slice the panettone into thick slices and butter each slice. Arrange the buttered panettone slices in an ovenproof dish. Scatter with the apple and sprinkle with a pinch of nutmeg. Pour over the cream mixture and make sure the panettone is evenly soaked. Sprinkle the top with brown sugar.

Place in the oven for 20 to 30 minutes or until golden and crispy.

SERVES 10

600ml/2½ cups of single/light cream

450ml/1¾ cups of milk

3 large eggs

1 vanilla pod/bean

150g/½ cup of caster/superfine sugar

1 panettone

Butter, for spreading

1 apple, peeled and finely diced

A pinch of nutmeg

50g/¼ cup of soft brown sugar

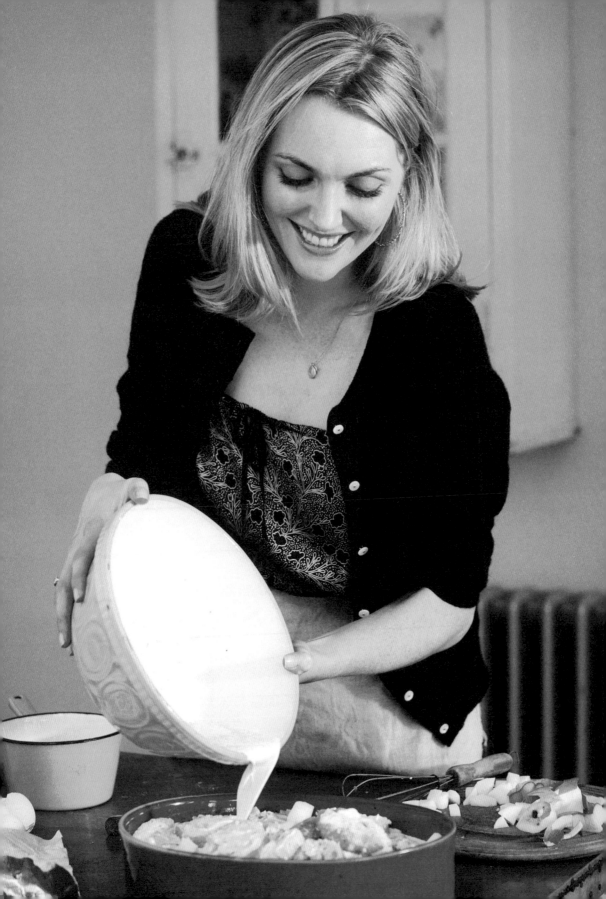

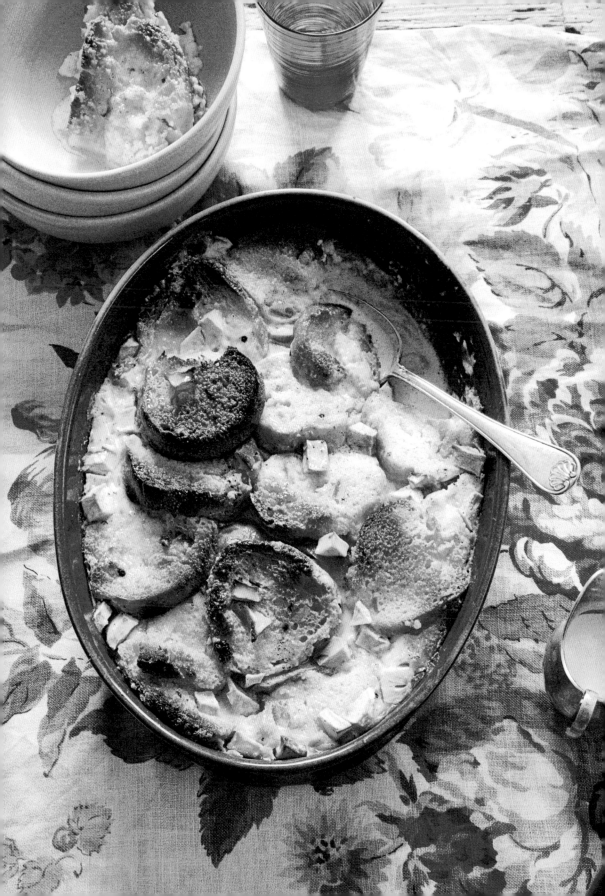

Coconut sorbet

SERVES 2–4

150g/generous ½ cup of
   caster/superfine sugar
125ml/½ cup of coconut
   milk
Juice of ½ a lime
40g/½ cup of desiccated
   coconut

This is up there with the Pineapple and Mint Granita for me. You can skip the lime if you are not a fan, but it gives it a lovely sharp edge.

Place the sugar in a heavy-bottomed pan. Add 185 to 250ml/¾ to 1 cup of water and simmer for 5 minutes, making a syrup. Stir in the coconut milk and lime juice. Add the desiccated coconut and allow the mixture to cool.

Churn in your ice-cream maker/sorbet machine as per the instructions. If you do not have an ice-cream maker, freeze the mixture in a plastic container for 2 hours. Remove from the freezer, pour into a blender and whiz for a minute or two. Pour back into the container. Freeze for another 2 hours, then serve.

Ruby Frais strawberry semifreddo

This recipe is so titled for a young girl named for a future of all things sweet, a Miss Ruby Frais. Her dad calls her 'Pudding' and she, like me, is partial to berries and vanilla ice cream. This then, quite literally, has her name all over it.

Put the strawberries in a bowl. Tip the sugar on top and leave to macerate for 1 hour. When they're a lovely, sticky mess, pour into a blender with the lemon juice and purée.

In a large bowl, whip the cream until thick but malleable enough to fall from the spoon. Pour the fruit into the cream and fold through thoroughly.

Put into an old ice-cream container or a loaf tin. Freeze for about 1 hour until crystals form around the edges, then take out and run through the blender. Freeze for 2 hours; blend again, then freeze for around 4 hours.

Take out 20 minutes before serving, slice and scatter over the meringues and some extra strawberries.

SERVES 4

450g/1lb of strawberries, hulled and halved, plus extra for serving

100g/¾ cup of icing/confectioners' sugar

Juice of ½ a small lemon

300ml/1¼ cups of double/heavy cream

30g/1oz of meringues, bashed up

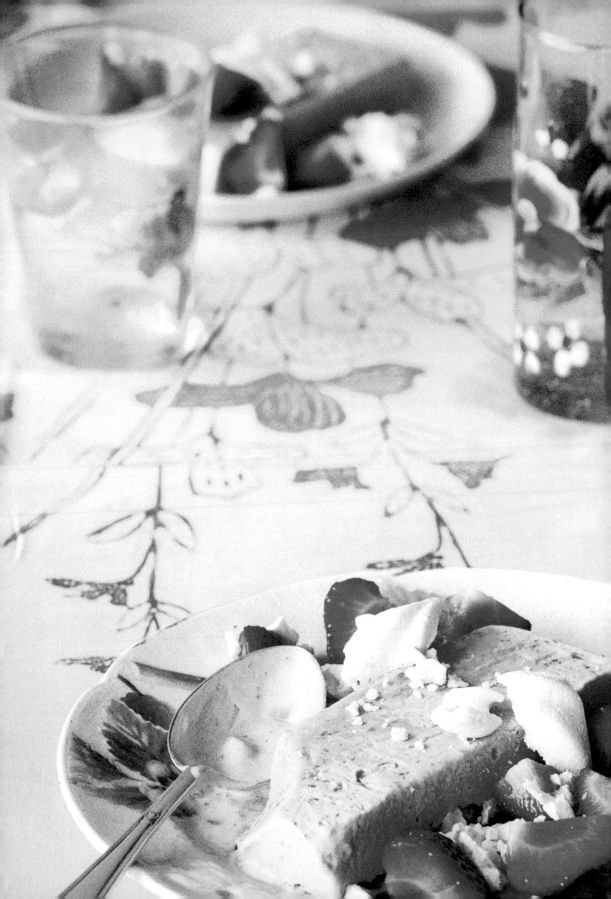

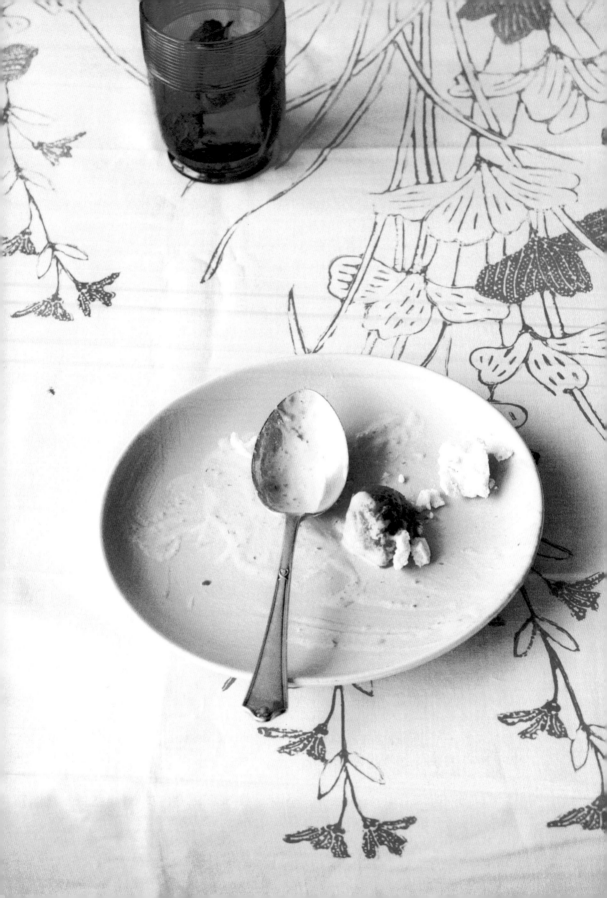

The Nutcracker

I wrote this story for Waitrose Food Illustrated magazine to go with a Christmas Syllabub recipe that I written for a December issue. They asked me to write a modern take on the Nutcracker and gave me quite a small word count in which to do it.

Here it is – I hope you like it.

It was Christmas Eve. In a spindly house perched in a row of other spindly houses, a girl with moist sugar plum eyes sat in a soft green chair. Her legs were thrown over the side, her shoes were scarlet ending in a rapier heel, and much to her mother's despair, if you squinted, you could see her knickers.

'Oh Maude.' The mother said. 'When will you sit like a lady?'

'My heart is broken.' Maude said. 'I will be ladylike when, and IF, I meet a MAN.'

'Is this about that boy?' Maude's father groaned.

'The King Rat?' Her little brother, Frederick asked. 'The one who snogged your friend Maxine at the dance?'

'Would you like to put the fairy on the top of the tree?' Her mother said.

'Don't bother me with your pagan trifles. My heart is broken.'

'Maude darling, do try and pull yourself together, your godfather will be here any minute. It's Christmas Eve. There will be many other boys. Could you try and summon a smile?'

Maude grimaced. The doorbell rang.

'Merry Christmas one and all!' Her godfather, M. Sousedalot, spun into the room on a sharp whisky breeze, his sandpaper voice grating the edges of Maude's misery.

'Frederick, for you dear, fat boy, a chocolate orange. And ah, Miss Heartbreak, for you, this – symbolic under the circumstances…'

It was a nutcracker.

'Uh, yeah, thanks?' Maude looked at her mother in appeal.

Fat Frederick (who wasn't normally allowed E numbers) ate his entire chocolate orange and got hyperactive.

'I want that nut man!' He said. 'Mum, my present's gone and Maude still has hers.'

He tried to snatch the nutcracker from Maude and, in the tussle, it slipped from his hot buttery hand. There was a crack as the nutcracker hit the floor. Half of his leg lay splintered beside him.

'Wow, Frederick. Has mum ever told you you're adopted?' Maude said.

After everyone had gone to bed, Maude lay under the Christmas tree listening to Wham's greatest hits, with the nutcracker in her hand. The King Rat had told her she was post-modern after he kissed her at The Fleet Foxes gig. What use post-modernism when she was alone under the mistletoe? She wondered. She shut her eyes. The clock chimed.

Shadows danced in her eyelids. Stealthy shadows wearing bosomy dresses and whispering, 'Look at Maude! She's so innocent and dull! Pick me, pick me.'

Maude opened her eyes and was greeted by an army of dancing rats in skinny jeans. Their horrible two-step was led by The King Rat himself, leering at her over Maxine's fake tanned shoulder. Dry ice swirled around them.

'Alright Maude.' He said.

'Go away!' Maude cried.

Closer and closer they came, until she could smell Maxine's cheap perfume and see the angry cluster of spots beading The King Rat's whiskers.

'I never really liked you.' Maxine said.

'Please leave me alone.' Maude begged.

She heard the sound of creaking wooden joints. Through the dry ice she saw a red uniform, a beard, a tall black hat.

'Allow me.' The Nutcracker said.

He marched through the dry ice, sending the rats scuttling in his wake. He felled The King Rat with one wooden blow. He hadn't bargained for Maxine though. She pulled out a bottle of hairspray from her bag and sprayed him squarely in the eyes. The Nutcracker stumbled drunkenly. Maude ran to him. As Maxine advanced, Maude took off her shoe and threw it at Maxine's beehive. It sliced through the middle like an arrow.

'My hair! You've ruined my hair.' Maxine shrieked and fainted clean away.

Maude led The Nutcracker through the fog, holding his hand as the darkness enveloped them. Until…

There was snow; everywhere there was snow and light. Maude turned to The Nutcracker, whose flesh-and-blood hand she realized she was holding. The beard and vice-tight jaw had melted somehow, revealing laughing eyes and a clean (and distinctly rugged) jaw.

'Wow.' Maude said, for the second time that night.

'Long story, involving a curse.' The Nutcracker said. 'Anyway, you've broken it, you goddess.'

They had arrived at a shimmering sea, on which a boat bobbed towards them. The Nutcracker picked Maude up and flung her in. She braced herself, but landed on a nest of rose-scented, belly-rounded softness.

'But it's Turkish Delight!' Maude's eyes were round.

The icebergs they wove between were meringues; glossy and soft peaked. Dark chocolate seals slipped beneath the boat and chased each other. They sailed forth through geysers of thick, sweet cream and rock pools of salted caramel. Their compass was a sugar plum mermaid, her tail a beacon, leading them home…

'Maude, when I said you'd meet other boys, I didn't mean now this instant, under the Christmas tree!' It was morning. Maude's mother stood above her, looking dangerous.

'What?!' Maude woke in the drowsy embrace of a man in red uniform.

'Madam, I can explain everything.' The Nutcracker said. 'In the mean time – Turkish Delight?'

Armagnac apricot pannacotta

SERVES 4

2 sheets of gelatine

500ml/2 cups of
   double/heavy cream

100g/½ cup of
   caster/superfine sugar

1 vanilla pod/bean, insides
   scraped

1 tablespoon of Armagnac

For the apricot compote

A small handful of dried
   apricots

125ml/½ cup of orange
   juice

1 tablespoon of Armagnac

1 tablespoon of
   caster/superfine sugar

Pannacotta is basically baked cream. No one said it was good for you, but God, it's good. I am a huge Armagnac fan. It works wonderfully tarting up dried fruit – apricots, prunes and plums – and it tastes very grown-up.

First, soak the gelatine sheets in some cold water. They should be soft after about 10 minutes. In a saucepan, mix together the cream, sugar and vanilla pod/bean and bring to a simmer, but not a boil. Remove from the heat and add the gelatine, mixing well. Add the Armagnac, mix and divide the mixture into four moulds. Refrigerate for at least 4 hours.

Whilst the pannacottas are setting, make an apricot compote. Place the apricots in a saucepan with the orange juice, Armagnac and sugar, stir and cook on low for 5 to 8 minutes. Keep to one side.

When you are about serve, take the pannacottas out of the fridge. Place the moulds in a shallow basin of warm water, coming up to halfway, and then turn out onto a serving dish and serve surrounded by the apricots.

Christmas sugar plum syllabubby mess

For charming men in uniform
Or, for charming men, in uniform.

Start with the meringues. Preheat the oven to its lowest setting and line a baking tray with non-stick baking/parchment paper. In a very clean, dry bowl, whisk the egg whites until they reach firm peaks. Gradually mix in the sugar and salt until the mixture is a thick cloud of white. This should take somewhere around 8 minutes, and an electric mixer is a blessing unless you are very staunch.

Spoon the mixture into eight rounds on the baking/parchment paper and bake for 1 hour 15 minutes or so, until firm but not highly coloured. Leave the meringues on a wire rack to cool.

To make the compote and syllabub, put the fruit in a small saucepan with about 60ml/¼ cup of water and the honey or agave on a low heat. Cook the fruit for around 8 minutes or until it has softened. Sieve, and set the fruit aside.

Put the juice back in the pan with the sugar on a low heat to make a syrup. This will take about 10 minutes. Reserve and cool. Chill the fruit for at least 1 hour.

Whisk together the cream with a few tablespoons of the reserved fruit syrup. When the mixture begins to thicken, add the Greek yoghurt and whisk some more. Now for the imaginative bit. Do you want individual servings or one big platter of meringues, with the fruit compote spooned on top and the cream and syrup spooned on top after that? Or, do you want to serve it in layers in individual coloured glasses, with some toasted almonds on top? Picture the land of sweets, and go for it...

MAKES 8

For the meringues
6 large egg whites
340g/1⅓ cups of
    caster/superfine sugar
A pinch of salt

For the rest
4 plums (about 250g/9oz),
    stoned and roughly
    chopped
4 pears, peeled, cored and
    roughly chopped
4 tablespoons of runny
    honey or agave syrup
3 tablespoons of
    caster/superfine sugar
185ml/¾ cup of
    double/heavy cream
185ml/¾ cup of Greek
    yoghurt
50g/½ cup of toasted
    flaked almonds

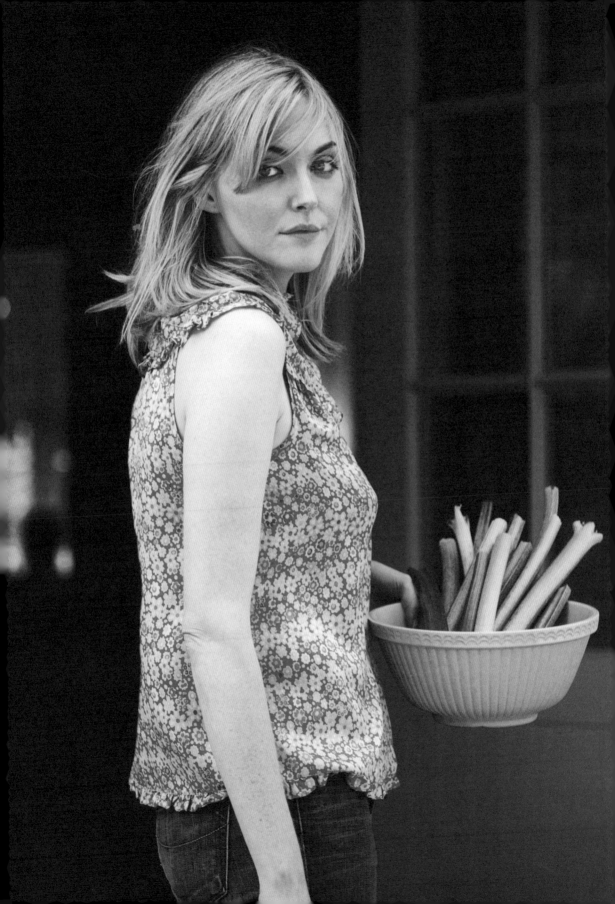

Acknowledgements and resounding thanks

My darling husband Jamie, you are everything that is good and right in the world. One day I will make poached eggs as beautifully as you do. Probably not though and breakfast wouldn't be half as fun.

My gorgeous family, pre-existing and the in-laws. Thank you for your recipes, stories and sweetness, and for your abiding love. Clover and Luke, thank you for all the many fantasy food games through the years and thank you for the daily debriefs. Ned, thank you for being such a demon onion chopper. Benji, thank you for chickens cottaging, pregnant caretaking, chauffeuring and happily sharing chocolate with me on the sofa whilst your brother is away. You rock.

A massive thank you to the food goddesses that continue to inspire and awe, sharing techniques, recipes and wisdom – Tiffany Crouch, Ginny Rolfe, and Alice Hart, you are all brilliant and I thank each one of you.

To the entire team at HarperCollins who make my life lovely and continue to make it all a pleasure. A huge thank you and big fat kiss to my wonderful editor Carole Tonkinson, Belinda Budge, Helen Hawksfield, Lee Motley and Anna Gibson for her enduring kindness, humour and attention to detail.

Thank you as ever to the creative team, to Jan Baldwin for your incredible photographs, skill and fun; Patrick Budge for your seamless design and dead lions in the garden; Alice Hart for beauteous food, chatting and morning sickness skills; Emma Thomas for your splendid props and eye; and Peter Dixon for being an all round gent.

Thank you dear Grainne Fox for your unerring support, sagacity, and ability to sort things out, and a big hug and thank you to Mink Choi.

Thank you Angela Becker for getting it from the beginning and having unbelievable patience and resolve. Thank you AND a squeeze to Catrina Naylor, fellow tour widow and logistics whizz.

My girlfriends – as always – thank you and much, much love.

SD

index

Suppliers

Porcelain tableware: Billy Lloyd, www.billylloyd.co.uk
Ceramic tableware: Toast, www.toast.co.uk
Vintage napkins: The Cloth Shop, www.theclothshop.net
Garden table: Petersham Nurseries, www.petershamnurseries.com
Cressida Bell woodland fabric: Borderline, www.borderlinefabrics.com
Floral rococo fabric: Mulberry Home, www.mulberryhome.com
Flowers: Scarlet and Violet, www.scarletandviolet.co.uk

The author and publisher would like to thank Rowley Leigh and Le Café Anglais for permission to include their recipe for Parmesan custard with anchovy toast and also Trina Hahnemann for the recipe Rye cracker breads with horseradish and smoked trout pâté.

Sophie Dahl began her career as a model, but writing was always her first love. In 2003 she wrote an illustrated novella called *The Man with the Dancing Eyes*, which was a *Times* bestselling book. This was followed by a novel, *Playing with the Grown-ups*, published to widespread praise by Bloomsbury in 2007. Dahl is a contributing editor at British *Vogue*. She has also written for, amongst others, *US Vogue*, *Waitrose Food Illustrated* magazine, the *Observer*, the *Guardian* and the *Saturday Times Magazine*.

A devoted eater and cook, she wrote a book which chronicled her misadventures with food, *Miss Dahl's Voluptuous Delights*, published by HarperCollins in 2009, which was her second *Times* bestseller. Following on the success of *Voluptuous Delights*, Dahl wrote and presented a popular BBC2 six-part cooking series, *The Delicious Miss Dahl*, which was sold to numerous countries all over the world.

Dahl lives in England where she continues to work on her journalism, fiction and baking.